Easy Air Fryer Seafood Recipes

The Simple and Quick way to cook Delicious Seafood-Based Recipes at home

By Donna Thomson

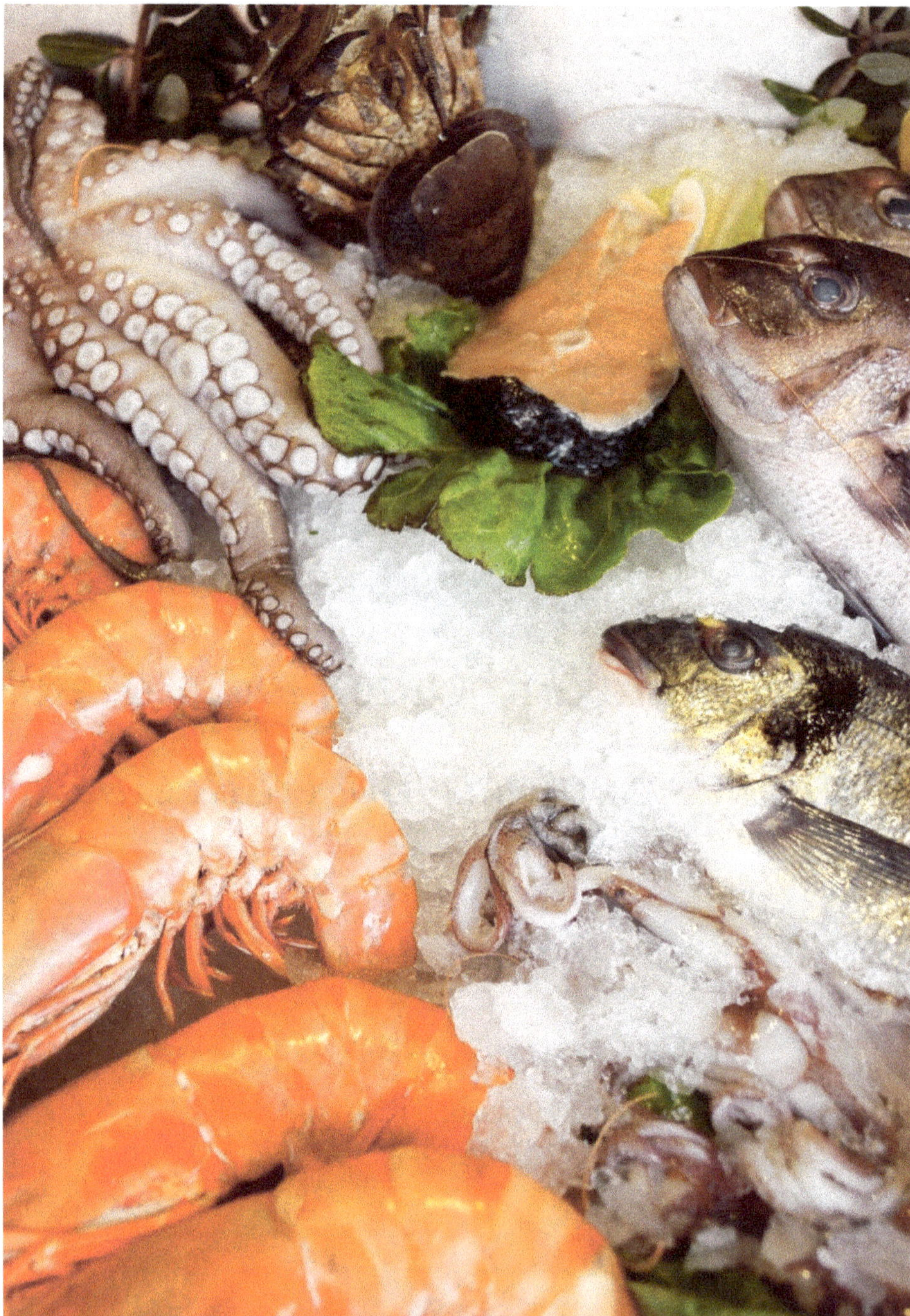

The content within this book has been derived from various sources. Please consult a licensed professional before attempting any techniques outlined in this book.

By reading this document, the reader agrees that under no circumstances is the author responsible for any losses, direct or indirect, which are incurred as a result of the use of information contained within this document, including, but not limited to, — errors, omissions, or inaccuracies.

Table of Contents

Air Fried Cod with Basil Vinaigrette

Serves: 4

Cooking Time: 15 minutes

Ingredients:

- ¼ cup olive oil /62.5ml
- 4 cod fillets
- A bunch of basil, torn
- Juice from 1 lemon, freshly squeezed
- Salt and pepper to taste

Instructions:

1) Warm up the air fryer for 5 minutes.
2) Sprinkle salt and pepper on the cod fillets.
3) Place in the air fryer and allow to cook for 15 at 3500 F or 177°C .
4) meanwhile, mix the other ingredients in a bowl and mix well to combine.
5) Serve the air fried cod using the basil vinaigrette.

Nutrition information:

- Calories per serving: 235

- Carbohydrates: 1.9g
- Protein: 14.3g
- Fat: 18.9g

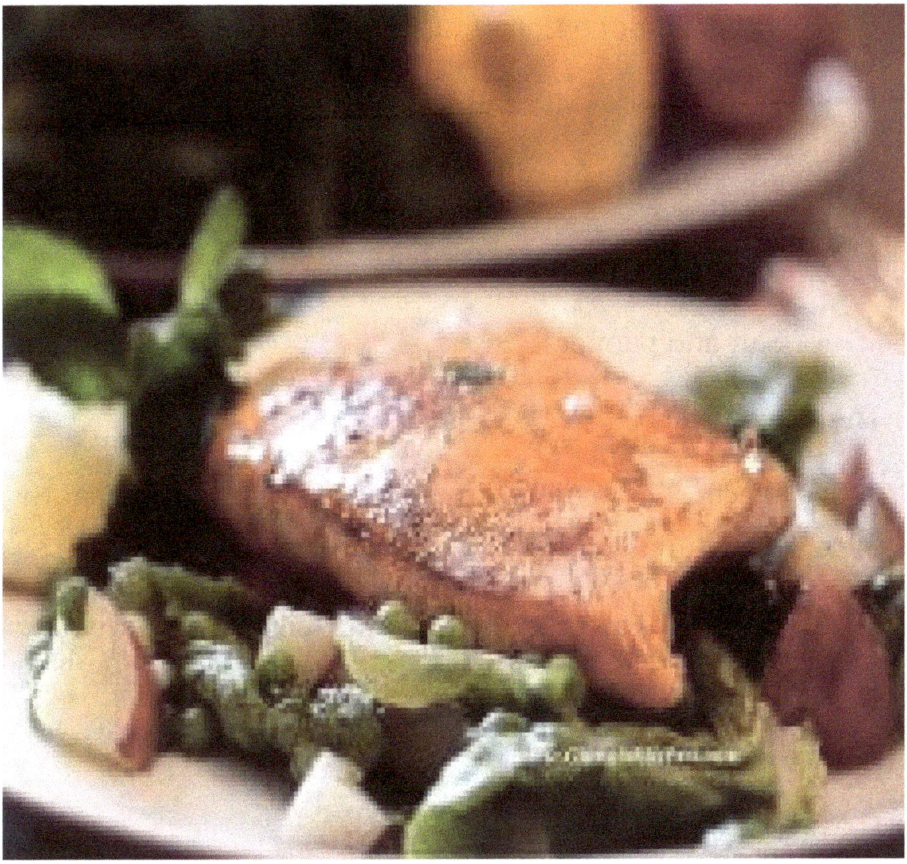

Almond Flour Coated Crispy Shrimps

Serves: 4

Cooking Time: 10 minutes

Ingredients:

- ½ cup almond flour /32.5g
- 1 tablespoon yellow mustard /15g
- 1-pound raw shrimps, peeled and deveined //450g
- 3 tablespoons olive oil /45ml
- Salt and pepper to taste

Instructions:

1) Place all ingredients in a Ziploc bag and shake vigorously to combine well.
2) Place the combined ingredients in a mid-air fryer and cook for 10 Minutes at 400°F or 205°C .

Nutrition information:

- Calories per serving: 206
- Carbohydrates: 1.3g
- Protein: 23.5g
- Fat: 11.9g

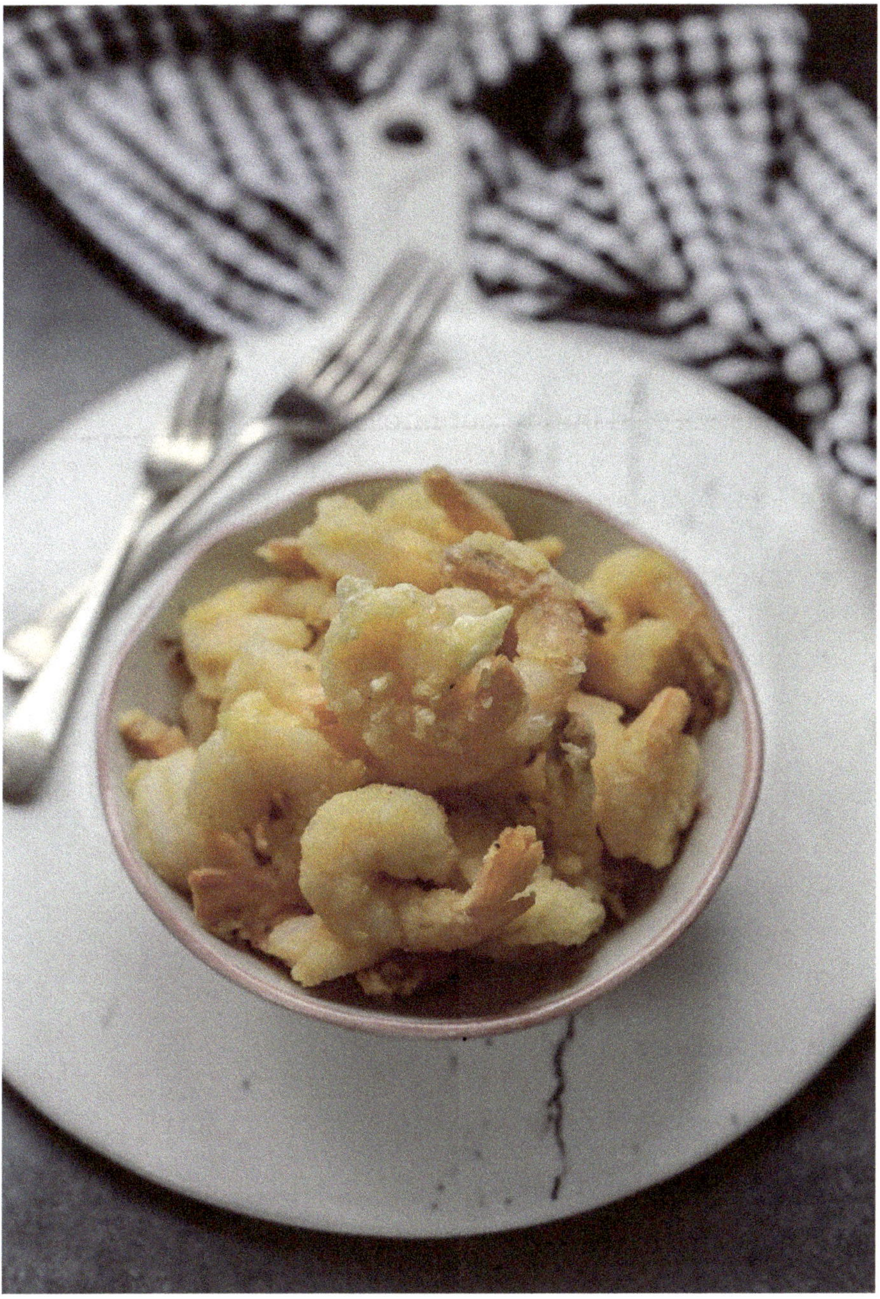

Another Crispy Coconut Shrimp Recipe

Servings per Recipe: 4

Cooking Time: 20

Ingredients:

- ½ cup flour /65g
- ½ stick cold butter, cut into cubes
- ½ tablespoon fresh lemon juice /7.5ml
- 1 egg yolk, beaten
- 1 green onion, chopped
- 1-pound salmon fillets, cut into small cubes /450g
- 3 tablespoons whipping cream /45ml
- 4 eggs, beaten

Salt and pepper to taste

Instructions:

1) Preheat your air fryer to 3900 F or 199°C.
2) Spice salmon fillets with lemon juice, salt and pepper to taste.

3) Mix the flour and butter in a bowl. Add cold water gradually while stirring to form a dough. Knead the dough into a sheet on a flat surface.

4) Place the dough in a baking pan, press the dough firmly in the baking pan.

5) Properly whisk the eggs and egg yolk in a bowl and season with salt and pepper to taste.

6) Place the salmon cubes on the baking pan lined with the dough and pour the whisked egg over it.

7) Cook for 15 to 20 minutes.

8) Dress with green onions once cooked.

Nutrition information:

- Calories per serving: 483
- Carbs: 5.2g
- Protein: 45.2g
- Fat: 31.2g

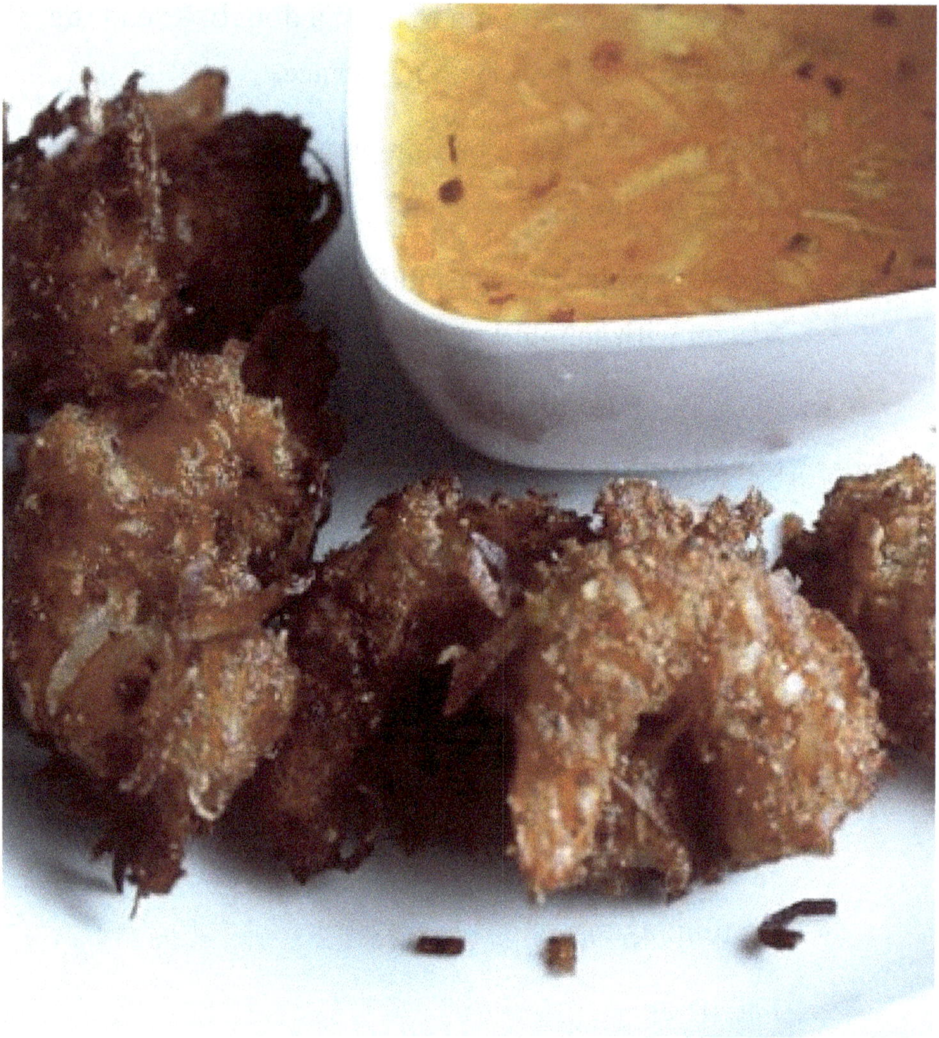

Apple Slaw Topped Alaskan Cod Filet

Servings per Recipe: 3

Cooking Time: 15

Ingredients:

- ¼ cup mayonnaise /62.5ml
- ½ red onion, diced
- 1 ½ pounds frozen Alaskan cod /675g
- 1 box wheat grains panko bread crumbs
- 1 granny smith apple, julienned
- 1 tablespoon vegetable oil /15ml
- 1 teaspoon paprika /5g
- 2 cups Napa cabbage, shredded /260g

Salt and pepper to taste

Instructions:

1) Preheat the air fryer to 3900 F or 199°C .
2) Place the grill pan accessory in the air fryer.
3) Brush some oil on the fish and place the fish in a bowl of breadcrumbs. Properly coat fish with breadcrumbs.

4) Place the fish in the grill pan and cook for seven and a half minutes, flip the fish and cook for an additional seven and a half minutes.

5) Meanwhile, prepare the slaw by mixing the residual Ingredients in the bowl.

6) Serve the fish with the slaw.

Nutrition information:

- Calories per serving: 316
- Carbs: 13.5g
- Protein: 37.8g
- Fat: 12.2g

Baked Cod Fillet Recipe From Thailand

Serves: 4

Cooking Time: 20 minutes

Ingredients:

- ¼ cup coconut milk, freshly squeezed /62.5ml
- 1 tablespoon lime juice, freshly squeezed /15ml
- 1-pound cod fillet, cut into bite-sized pieces /450g
- Salt and pepper to taste

Instructions:

1) Warm up your mid-air fryer for 5 minutes.
2) Place all ingredients in a baking pan.
3) Place the baking pan in the mid-air fryer.
4) Let it cook for 20 minutes at 3250 F or 163°C.

Nutrition information:

- Calories per serving: 844
- Carbohydrates: 2.3g
- Protein: 21.6g
- Fat: 83.1g

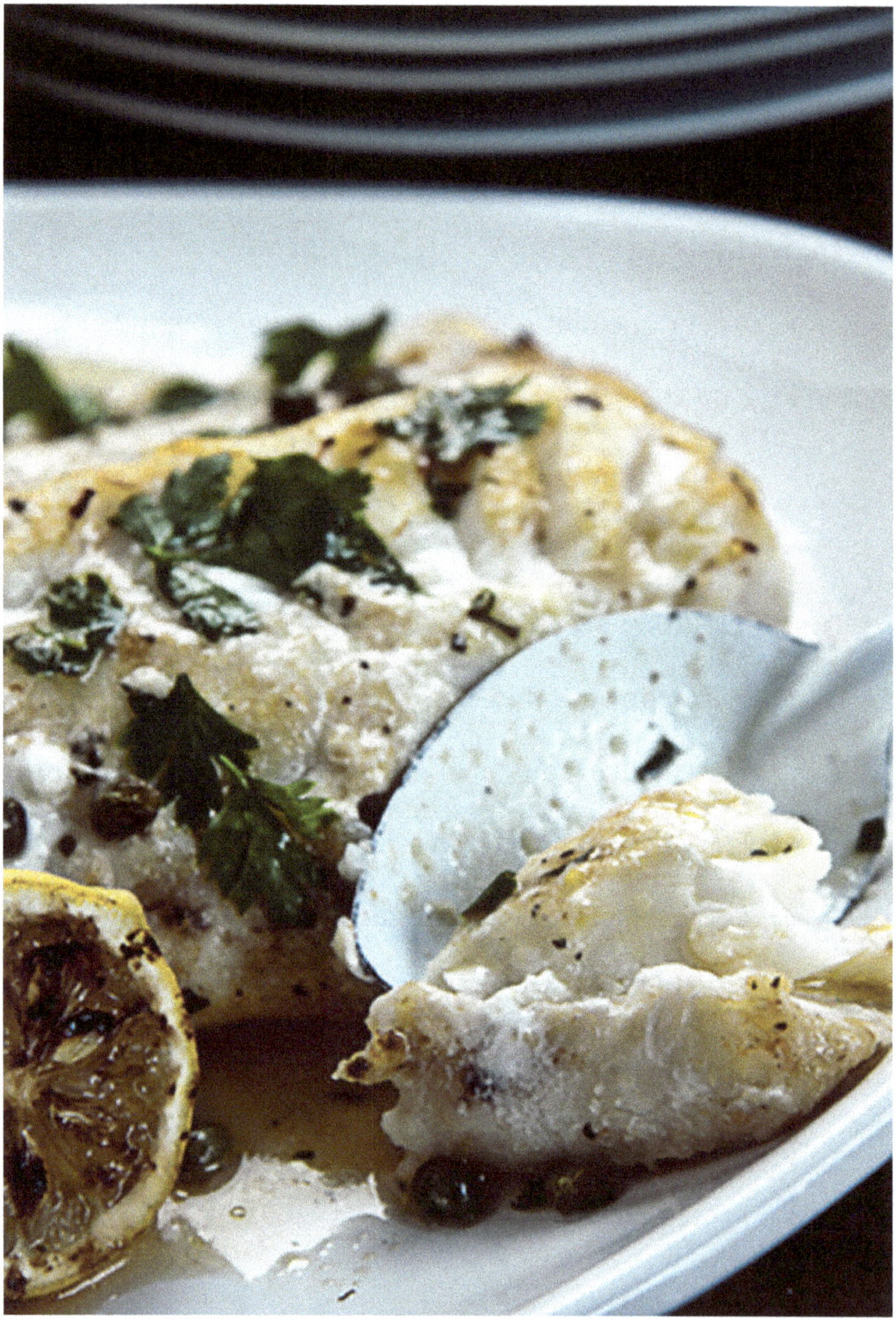

Baked Scallops with Garlic Aioli

Servings per Recipe: 4

Cooking Time: 10

Ingredients:

- 1 cup bread crumbs /130g
- 1/4 cup chopped parsley /32.5g
- 16 sea scallops, rinsed and drained
- 2 shallots, chopped
- 3 pinches ground nutmeg
- 4 tablespoons essential olive oil /60ml
- 5 cloves garlic, minced
- 5 tablespoons butter, melted /75ml
- Salt and pepper to taste

Instructions:

1) Lightly grease your baking pan with oil.
2) In a bowl, mix shallots, garlic, melted butter, and scallops. Season with pepper, salt, and nutmeg.
3) In another bowl, properly whisk organic olive oil and bread crumbs. Sprinkle over scallops.
4) Cook on 3900 F or 199°C for 10 minutes until lightly brown.
5) Dress with a sprinkle of parsley and serve.

Nutrition Information:

- Calories per Serving: 452
- Carbs: 29.8g
- Protein: 15.2g
- Fat: 30.2g

Basil ‘n Lime-Chili Clams

Servings per Recipe: 3

Cooking Time: 15 minutes

Ingredients:

- ½ cup basil leaves /65g
- ½ cup tomatoes, chopped /65g
- 1 tablespoon fresh lime juice /15ml
- 25 littleneck clams
- 4 cloves of garlic, minced
- 6 tablespoons unsalted butter /90g
- Salt and pepper to taste

Instructions:

1) Prewarm the air fryer to 3900 F or 199°C.
2) Place a fitting grill pan in the air fryer.
3) Place all ingredients in a large foil and fold over. Tuck the edges.
4) Place in a grill pan and cook for 15 minutes.
5) Serve with bread.

Nutrition information:

- Calories per serving: 163
- Carbs: 4.1g
- Protein: 1.7g

- Fat: 15.5g

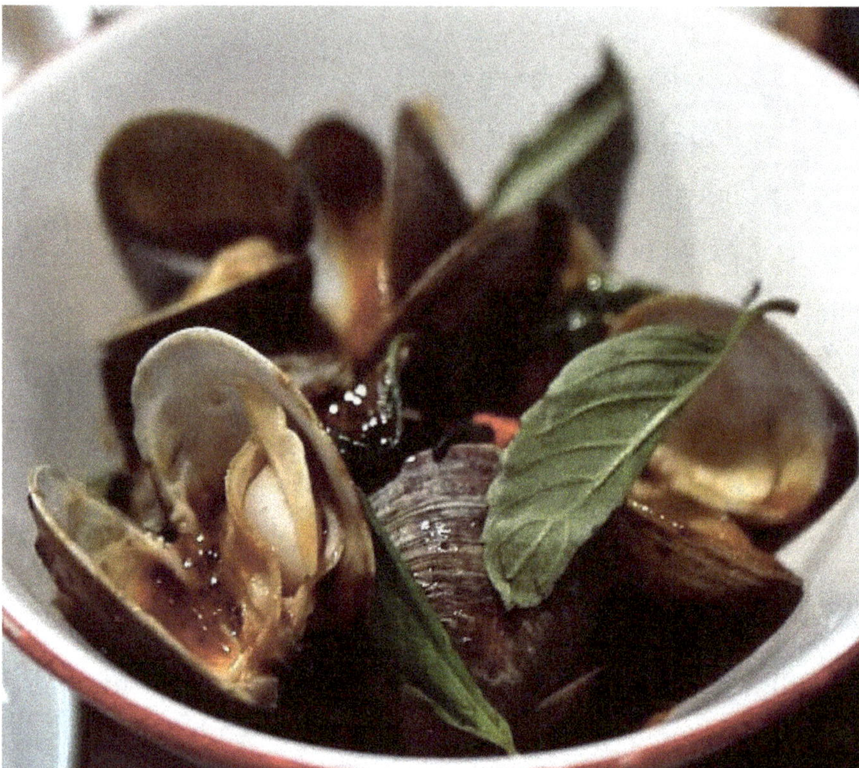

Bass Filet in Coconut Sauce

Serves: 4

Cooking Time: 15

Ingredients:

- ¼ cup coconut milk
- ½ pound bass fillet
- 1 tablespoon organic olive oil /15ml
- 2 tablespoons jalapeno, chopped /30g
- 2 tablespoons lime juice, freshly squeezed /30ml
- 3 tablespoons parsley, chopped /45g
- Salt and pepper to taste

Instructions:

1) Warm mid-air fryer for 5 minutes.
2) Spice the bass with salt and pepper to taste.
3) Brush the top with organic olive oil.
4) Place in the air fryer and cook for 15 at 3500 F or 177°C.
5) Meanwhile, in a saucepan, add coconut milk, lime juice, jalapeno and parsley.
6) Cook over medium heat.
7) Serve the fish with coconut sauce.

Nutrition information:

- Calories per serving: 139
- Carbohydrates: 2.7g
- Protein: 8.7g
- Fat: 10.3

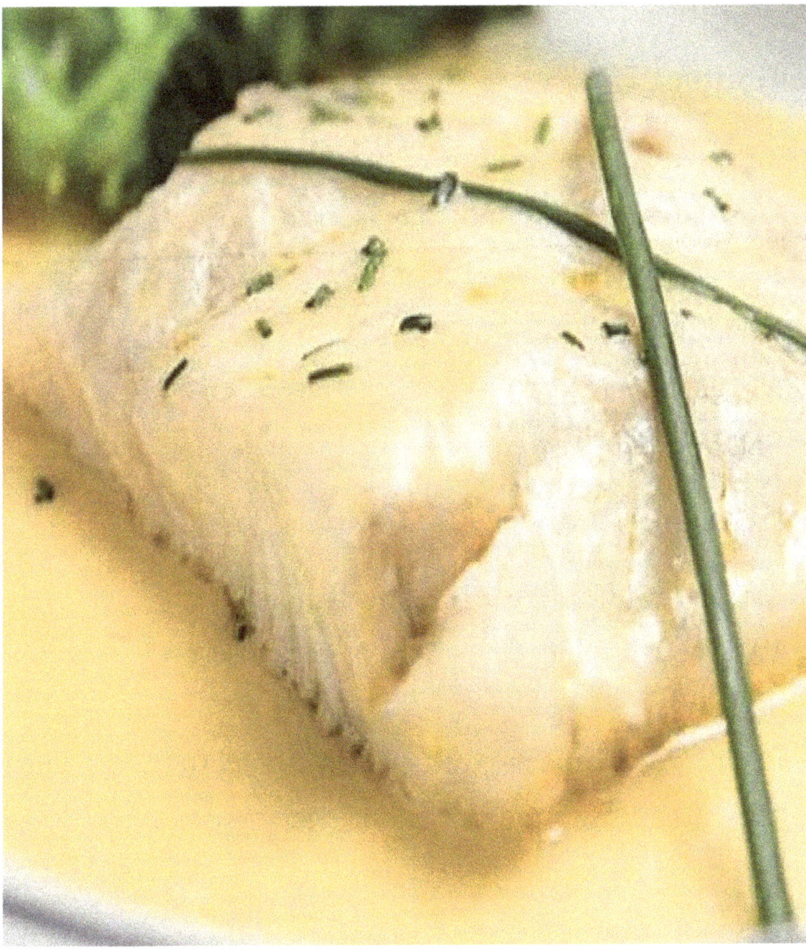

Beer Battered Cod Filet

Servings per Recipe: 2

Cooking Time: 15 minutes

Ingredients:

- ½ cup all-purpose flour /65g
- ¾ teaspoon baking powder /3.75g
- 1 ¼ cup lager beer /312.5ml
- 2 cod fillets
- 2 eggs, beaten
- Salt and pepper to taste

Instructions:

1) Preheat mid-air fryer to 3900 F or 199°C .
2) Pat the fish fillets dry with a paper towel and set them aside.
3) Combine all other ingredients in a bowl to form a batter.
4) Dip the fillets in the batter and place them in the double layer rack.
5) Cook for 15 minutes.

Nutrition information:

- Calories per serving: 229
- Carbs: 33.2g
- Protein: 31.1g

- Fat: 10.2g

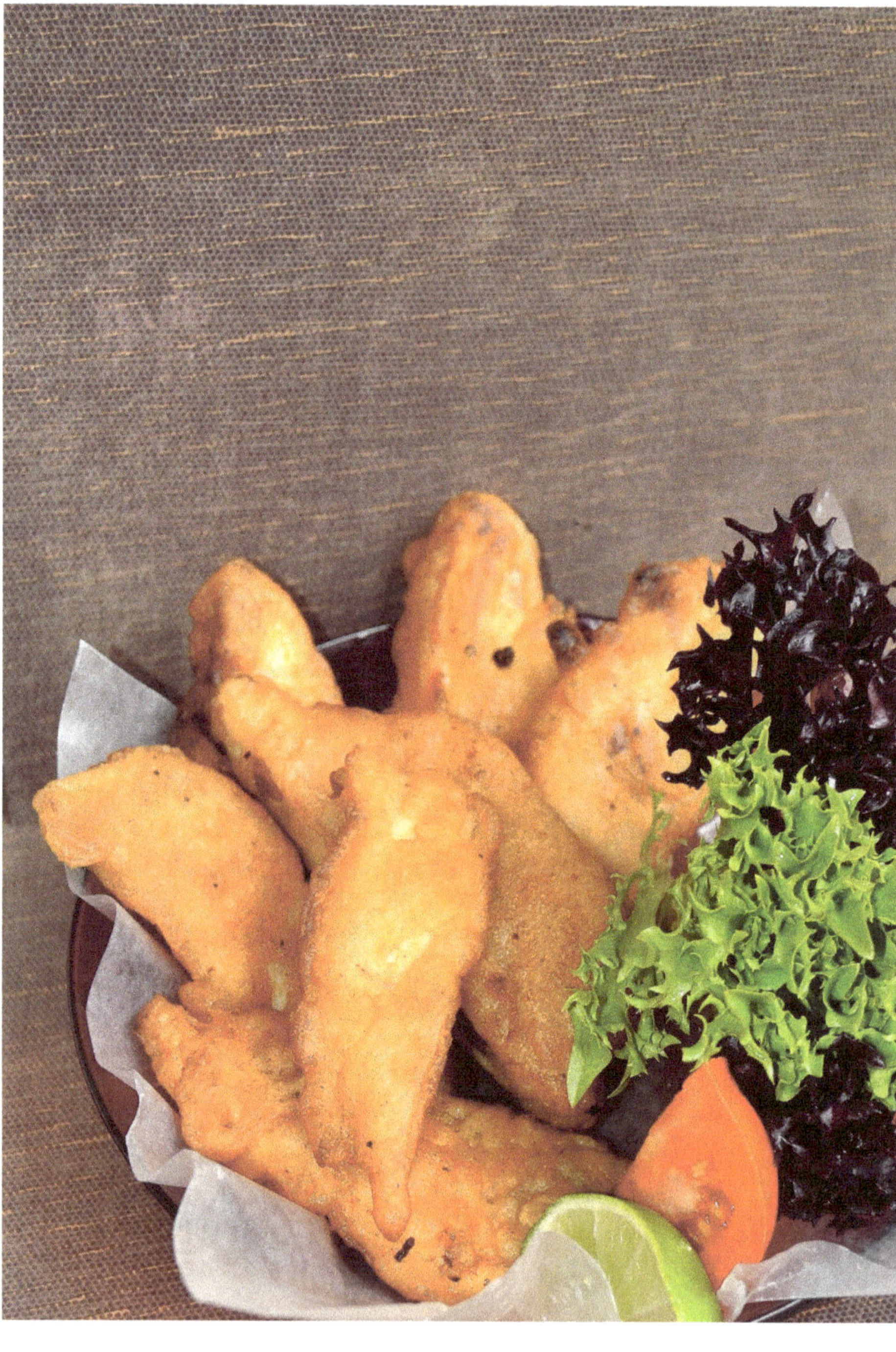

Buttered Baked Cod with Wine

Servings per Recipe: 2

Cooking Time: 12 minutes

Ingredients:

- 1 tablespoon butter /15g
- 1 tablespoon butter /15g
- 2 tablespoons dry white wine /30g
- 1/2 pound thick-cut cod loin /225g
- 1-1/2 teaspoons chopped fresh parsley /7.5g
- 1-1/2 teaspoons chopped green onion /7.5g
- 1/2 lemon, cut into wedges
- 1/4 sleeve buttery round crackers (for example Ritz®), crushed
- 1/4 lemon, juiced

Instructions

1) Put butter in a bowl, place in a microwave to melt and whisk in the crackers.
2) Lightly brush some butter in the baking pan. Place the baking pan in the air fryer and heat for two minutes at 3900 F or 199°C.
3) Grab a small bowl, mix lemon juice, white wine, parsley, and green onion. Whisk well to combine.

4) Dip the cod filets in melted butter. Pour the dressing on it. Add the butter-cracker mixture.
5) Cook for 10 Minutes at 3900 F or 199°C in the air fryer.
6) Serve with a dashing slice of lemon juice.

Nutrition Information:

- Calories per Serving: 266
- Carbs: 9.3g
- Protein: 20.9g
- Fat: 16.1g

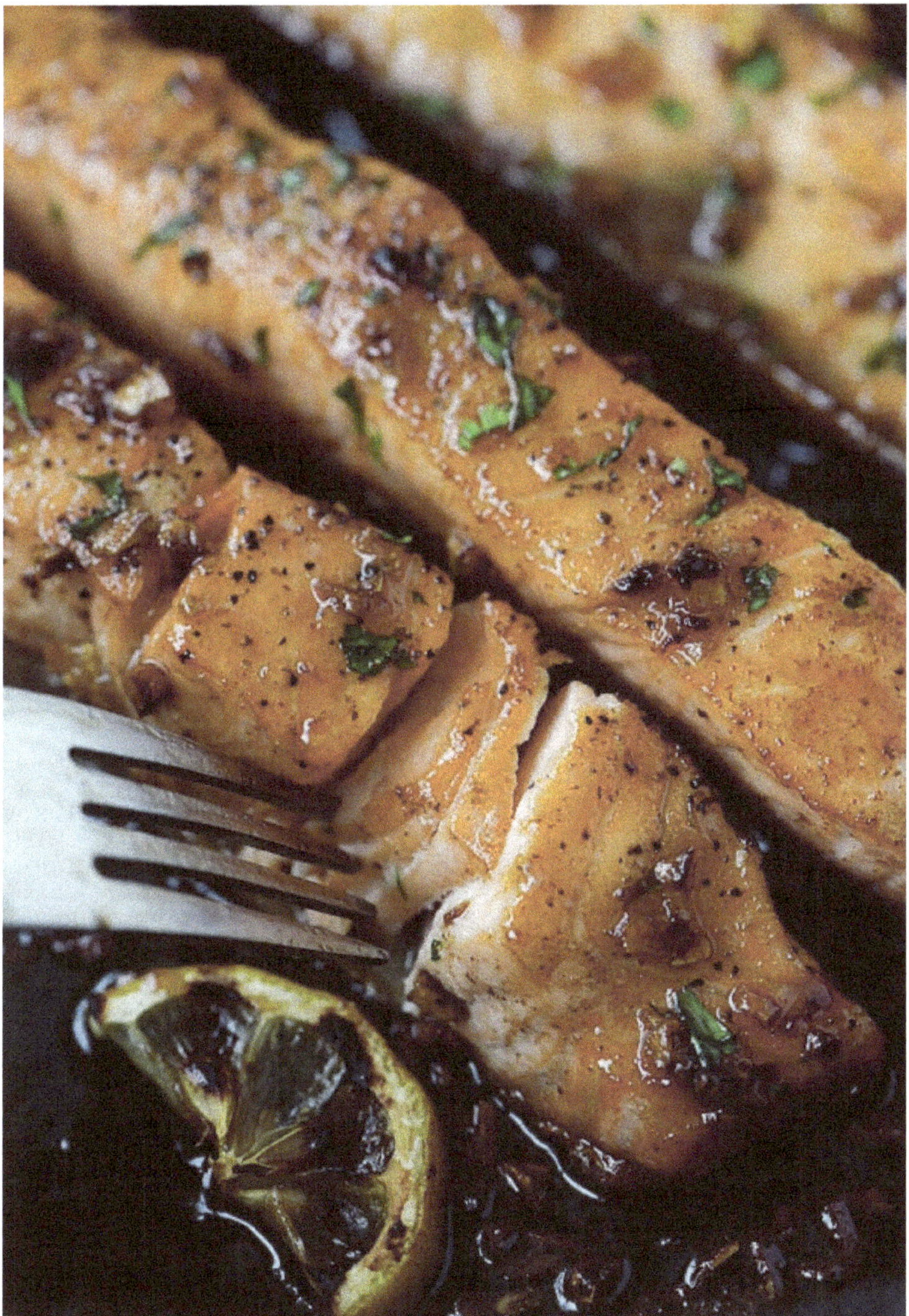

Buttered Garlic-Oregano on Clams

Servings per Recipe: 4

Cooking Time: 5 minutes

Ingredients:

- ¼ cup mozzarella, grated /32.5g
- ¼ cup parsley, chopped /32.5g
- 1 cup breadcrumbs /130g
- 1 teaspoon dried oregano /5g
- 2 dozen clams, shucked
- 3 cloves of garlic, minced
- 4 tablespoons butter, melted /60ml

Instructions:

1) While preheating your air fryer to 3900 F or 199°C add the breadcrumbs, parmesan cheese, parsley, oregano, and garlic in a medium-size bowl and stir in the melted butter.
2) Fill the baking pan with the clams.
3) Sprinkle the crumb mixture on the clams and place it in the air fryer.
4) Cook for 5 minutes.

Nutrition information:

- Calories per serving: 160

- Carbs: 6.3g
- Protein: 2.9g
- Fat: 13.6g

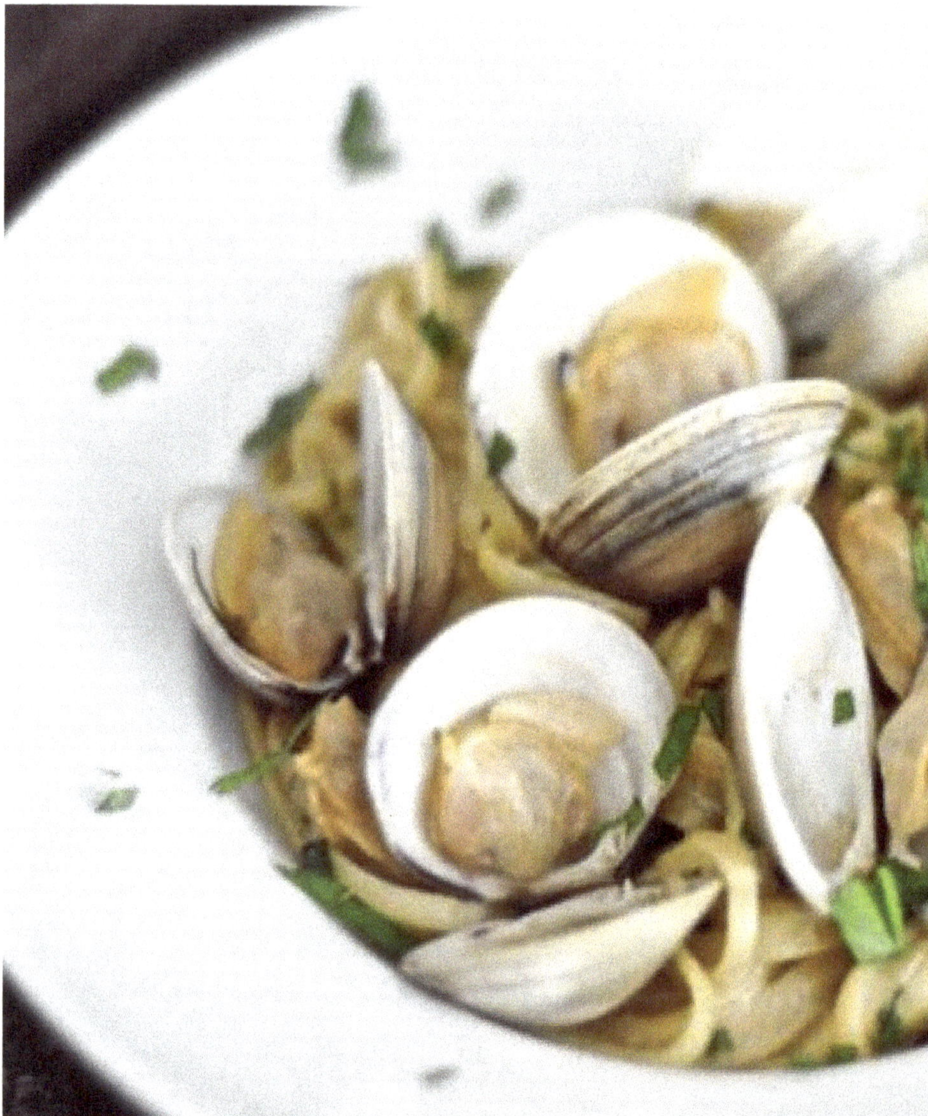

Butterflied Prawns with Garlic-Sriracha

Servings per Recipe: 2

Cooking Time: 15

Ingredients:

- 1 tablespoon lime juice /15ml
- 1 tablespoon sriracha /15g
- 1-pound large prawns, shells removed and cut lengthwise or butterflied /450g
- 1 teaspoon fish sauce /5ml
- 2 tablespoons melted butter /30ml
- 2 tablespoons minced garlic /30g
- Salt and pepper to taste

Instructions:

1) Preheat the air fryer to 3900 F or 199°C using the air fryer setting.
2) Place the grill pan in the mid-air fryer.
3) Spice the prawns with all other mentioned ingredients.
4) Place in the grill pan and cook for 15 minutes. Flip over halfway through cooking time.

Nutrition information:

- Calories per serving: 443
- Carbs:9.7 g

- Protein: 62.8g
- Fat: 16.9g

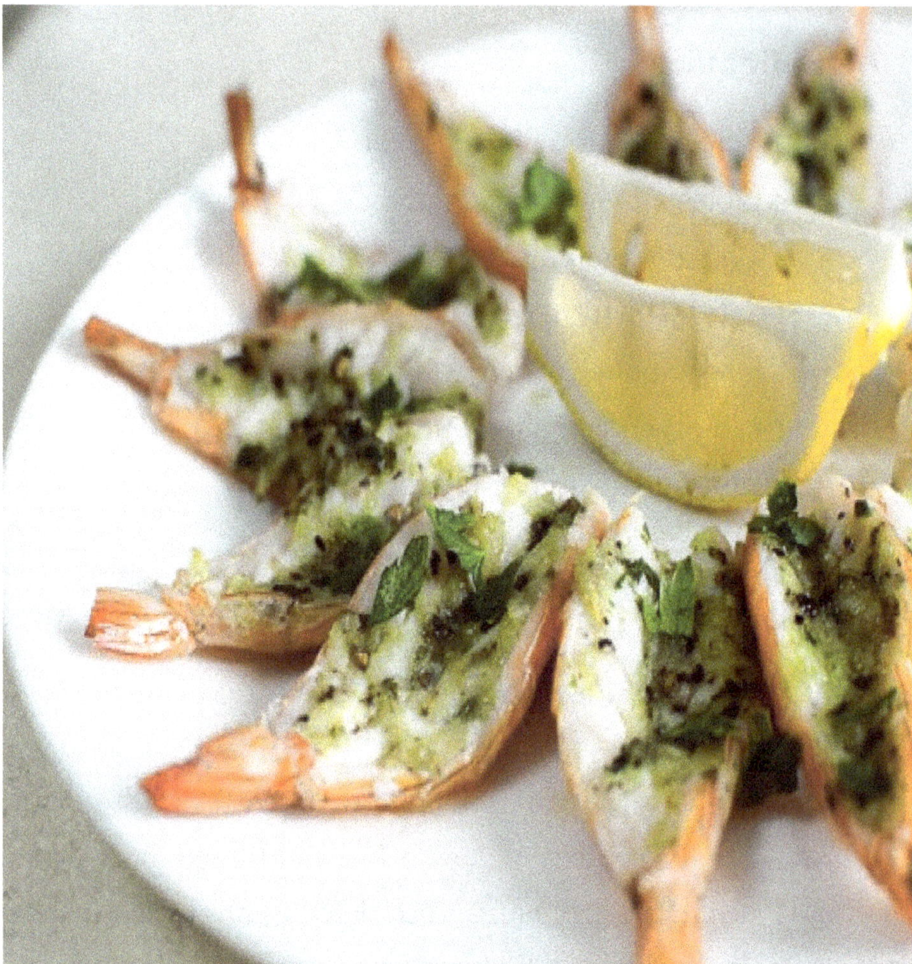

Cajun Seasoned Salmon Filet

Serves: 1

Cooking Time: 15

Ingredients:

- 1 salmon fillet
- 1 teaspoon juice from lemon, freshly squeezed /5ml
- 3 tablespoons extra virgin essential olive oil /45ml
- A dash of Cajun seasoning mix
- Salt and pepper to taste

Instructions:

1) Preheat the air fryer for 5 minutes using the air fryer setting.
2) Place all ingredients inside a bowl, mix well to coat.
3) Place the fish fillet in the air fryer's basket.
4) Bake for 15 minutes at 3250 F or 163°C .
5) Once cooked brush with extra virgin olive oil

Nutrition information:

- Calories per serving: 523
- Carbohydrates: 4.6g
- Protein: 47.9g
- Fat: 34.8g

Cajun Spiced Lemon-Shrimp Kebabs

Servings per Recipe: 2

Cooking Time: 10 minutes

Ingredients:

- 1 tsp cayenne /5g
- 1 tsp garlic powder /5g
- 1 tsp kosher salt /5g
- 1 tsp onion powder /5g
- 1 tsp oregano /5g
- 1 tsp paprika /5g
- 12 pcs XL shrimp
- 2 lemons, sliced thinly crosswise
- 2 tbsp extra virgin olive oil /30ml

Instructions:

1) Mix all ingredients except the lemons. Marinate for 10 minutes.
2) Fasten 3 shrimps on a steel skewer.
3) Place the above in a skewer rack.
4) Cook for 5 minutes at 3900 F or 199°C .
5) Squeeze lemon juice on the shrimps and serve.

Nutrition Information:

- Calories per Serving: 232

- Carbs: 7.9g
- Protein: 15.9g
- Fat: 15.1g

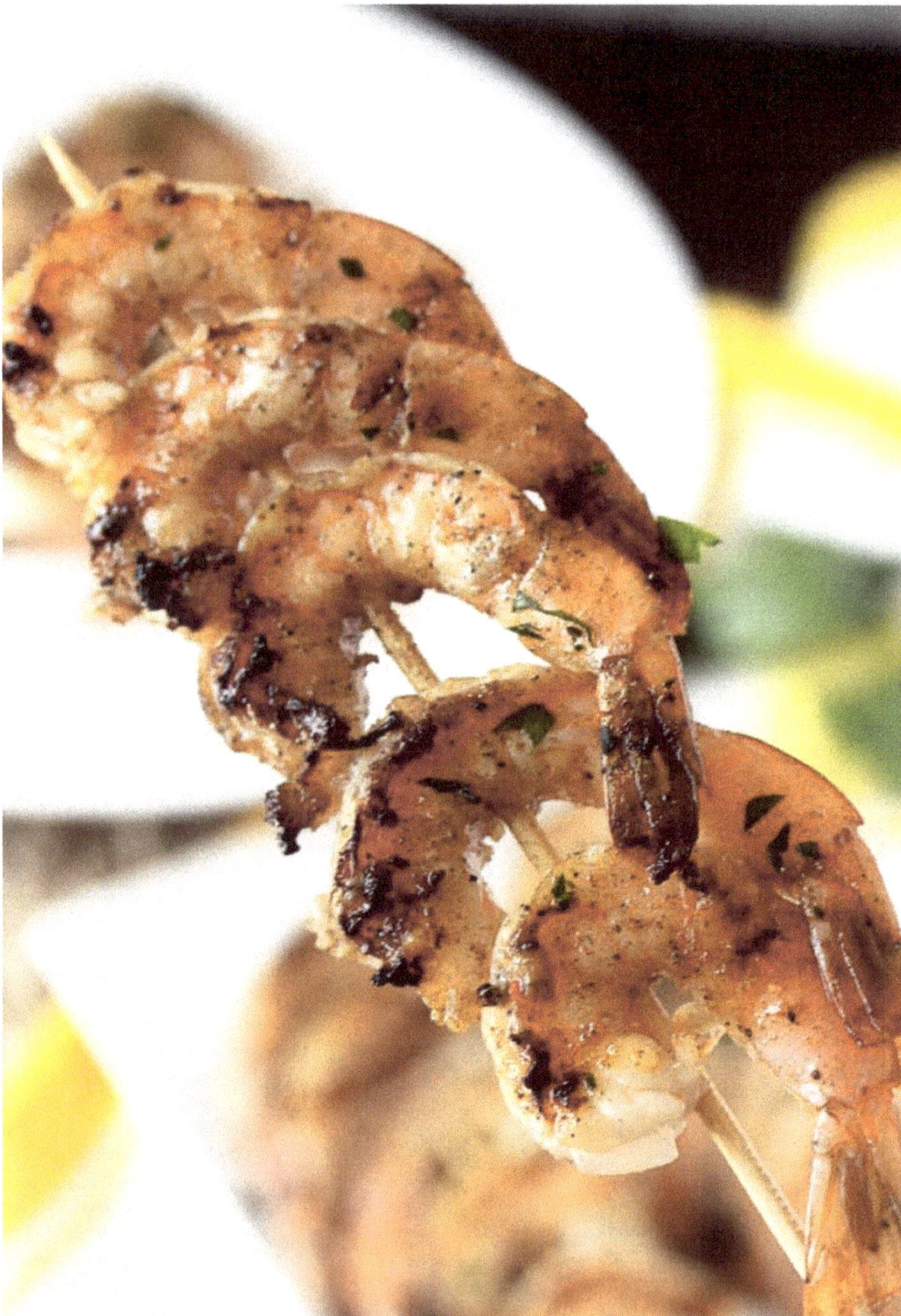

Cajun Spiced Veggie-Shrimp Bake

Servings per Recipe: 4

Cooking Time: 20 minutes

Ingredients:

- 1 Bag of Frozen Mixed Vegetables
- 1 Tbsp Gluten-Free Cajun Seasoning /15g
- Olive Oil Spray
- Season with salt and pepper
- Small Shrimp Peeled & Deveined (Regular Size Bag about 50-80 Small Shrimp)

Instructions:

1) With a cooking spray lightly grease a baking pan with any oil of your choice. Add all ingredients to the baking pan and stir well to coat. Season with pepper and salt to taste.
2) Cook on 3300 F or 166°C for 10 minutes. Stir after every 5 minutes.
3) Serve and enjoy.

Nutrition Information:

- Calories per Serving: 78
- Carbs: 13.2g
- Protein: 2.8g
- Fat: 1.5g

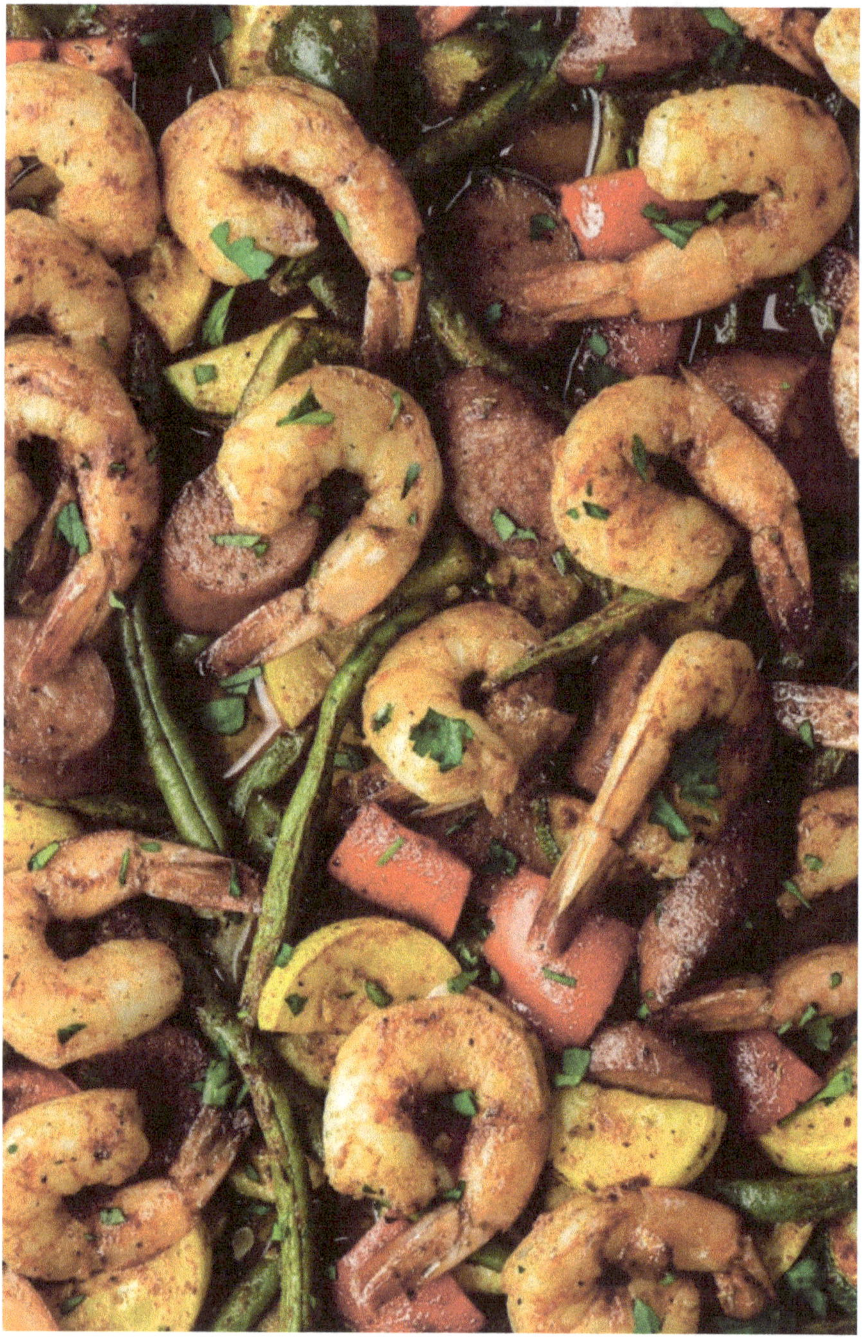

Celery leaves 'n Garlic-oil Grilled Turbot

Servings per Recipe: 2

Cooking Time: 20 minutes

Ingredients:

- ½ cup chopped celery leaves /65g
- 1 clove of garlic, minced
- 2 tablespoons olive oil /30ml
- 2 whole turbot, scaled and head removed
- Salt and pepper to taste

Instructions:

1) Preheat the air fryer to 3900 F or 199°C using the air fryer settings.
2) Place the grill pan in the air fryer.
3) Season the turbot with salt, pepper, garlic, celery leaves and then brush with oil.
4) Gently place in the grill pan and cook for 20 minutes until the fish becomes flaky

Nutrition information:

- Calories per serving: 269
- Carbs: 3.3g
- Protein: 66.2g
- Fat: 25.6g

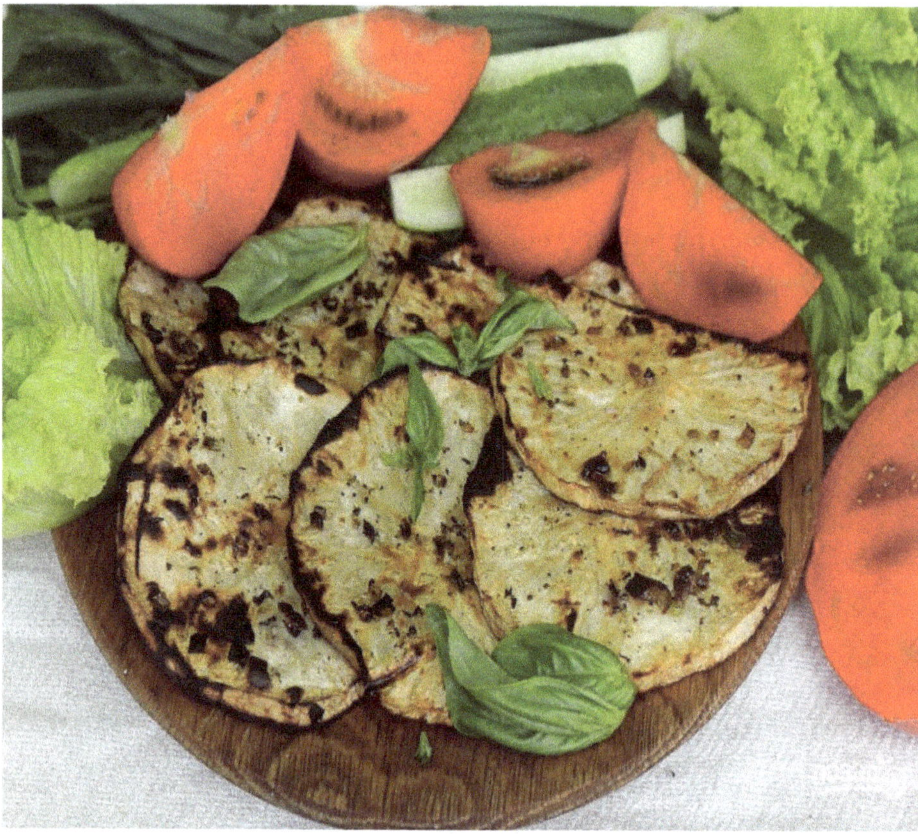

Char-Grilled Drunken Halibut

Servings per Recipe: 6

Cooking Time: 20 minutes

Ingredients:

- 1 tablespoon chili powder /15g
- 2 cloves of garlic, minced
- 3 pounds halibut fillet, skin removed /1350g
- 4 tablespoons dry white wine /60g
- 4 tablespoons olive oil /60ml
- Salt and pepper to taste

Instructions:

1) Put all ingredients in the large Ziploc bag.
2) Place in the fridge and allow to marinate for 2 hours.
3) Preheat the air fryer to 3900 F or 199°C .
4) Place the grill pan accessory in the air fryer.
5) Grill the fish for 20 minutes making sure to turn it over every 5 minutes.

Nutrition information:

- Calories per serving: 385
- Carbs: 1.7g
- Protein: 33g
- Fat: 40.6g

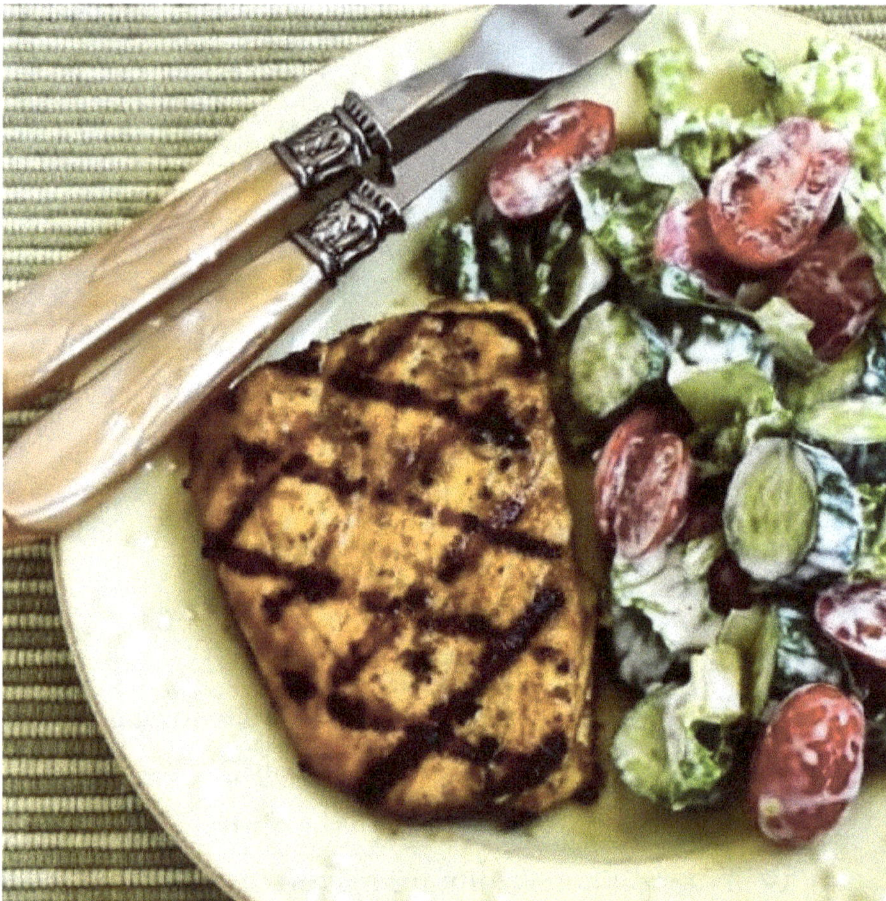

Clams with Herbed Butter in Packets

Servings per Recipe: 2

Cooking Time: 20 Minutes

Ingredients:

- ½ cup unsalted butter, diced /65g
- 1 tablespoon dill, chopped /15g
- 1 tablespoon fresh freshly squeezed lemon juice/15ml
- 1 tablespoon parsley, chopped /15g
- 24 littleneck clams, scrubbed clean
- Lemon wedges
- Salt and pepper to taste

Instructions:

1) Preheat mid-air fryer to 3900 F or 199°C .
2) Place the grill pan in the air fryer.
3) Place clams and other ingredients on a large foil. Fold the foil and wrap the edges.
4) Place on the grill pan and cook for 15 to 20 minutes or until all clams are opened.

Nutrition information:

- Calories per serving: 384
- Carbs: 6g
- Protein: 18g

- Fat: 32g

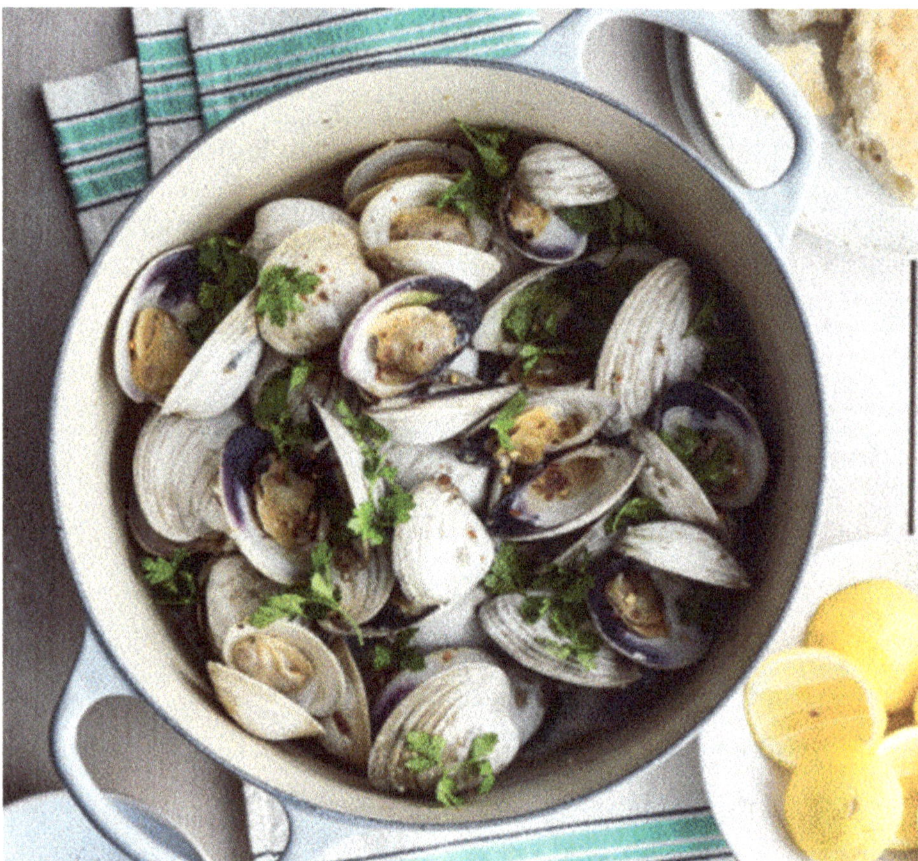

Cocktail Prawns in Air Fryer

Servings per Recipe: 1

Cooking Time: 8 minutes

Ingredients:

- ½ teaspoon black pepper /2.5g
- ½ teaspoon sea salt /2.5g
- 1 tablespoon ketchup /15ml
- 1 tablespoon white wine vinegar /15ml
- 1 teaspoon chili flakes /5g
- 1 teaspoon chili powder /5g
- 12 prawns, shelled and deveined

Instructions:

1) Preheat the air fryer to 390 o F or 199°C .
2) Place the shrimps in a bowl.
3) Stir in the other ingredients in a bowl. Coat shrimps with the content of the bowl.
4) Place the shrimps on the double layer rack and cook for 8 minutes.
5) Serve with mayonnaise (optional).

Nutrition information:

- Calories per serving: 148
- Carbs: 9.8g

- Protein: 21.9g
- Fat: 2.3g

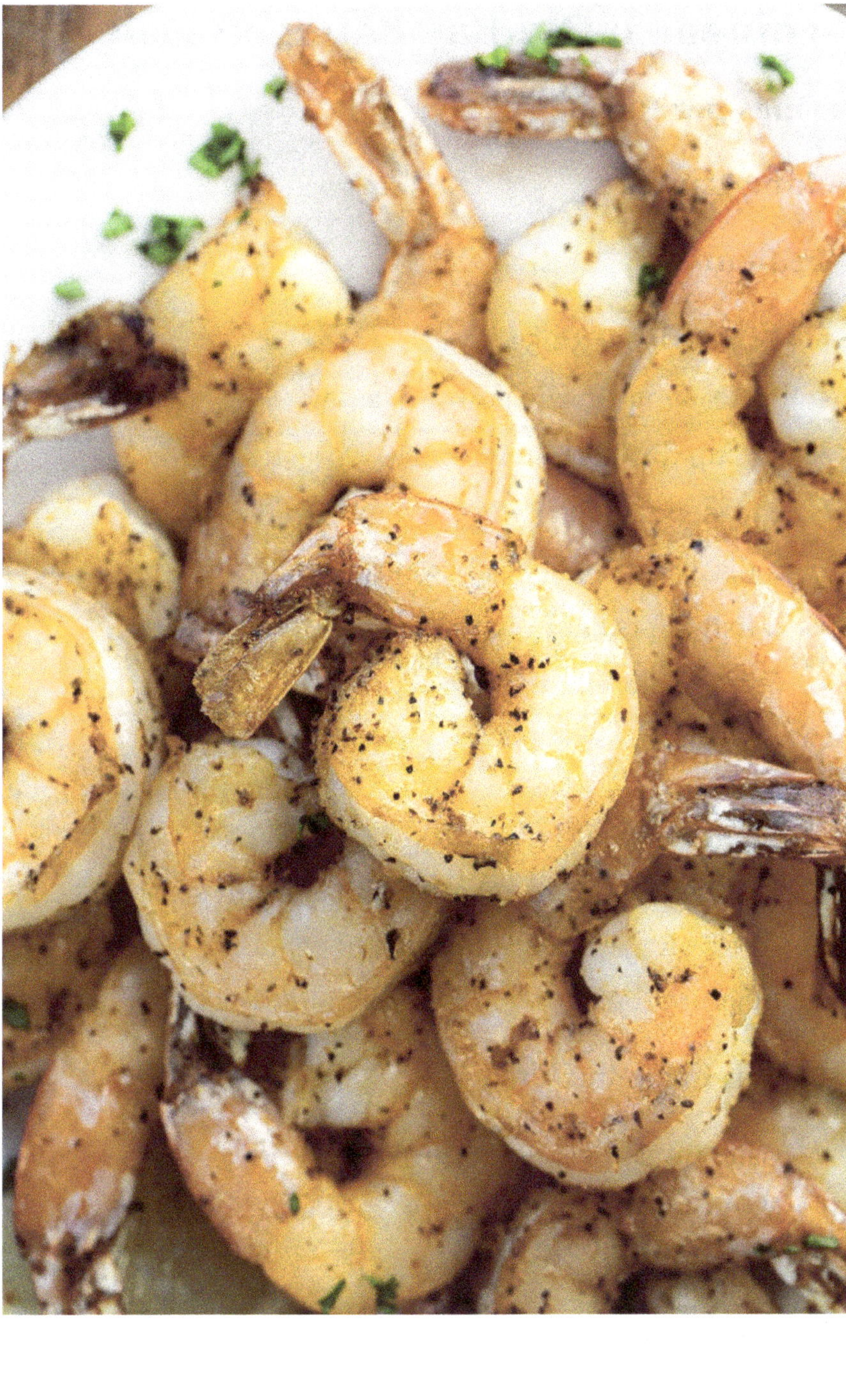

Cornmeal 'n Old Bay Battered Fish

Servings per Recipe: 6

Cooking Time: 15

Ingredients:

- ¼ cup flour /32.5g
- ½ teaspoon garlic powder /2.5g
- ¾ cup fine cornmeal /88g
- 1 teaspoon paprika /5g
- 2 teaspoons old bay seasoning /30g
- 6 fish fillets cut in half
- Salt and pepper to taste

Instructions:

1) Preheat the air fryer to 3300 F or 166°C .
2) In a Ziploc bag add the cornmeal, flour, seasonings, fish fillets and shake well for fish to coat.
3) Place on the double layer rack and cook for 15 minutes.

Nutrition information:

- Calories per serving: 239
- Carbs: 10.1g
- Protein: 22.9g
- Fat: 11.8g

Crisped Flounder Filet with Crumb Tops

Servings per Recipe: 4

Cooking Time: 15 minutes

Ingredients:

- 1 cup dry bread crumbs /130g
- 1 egg beaten
- 1 lemon, sliced
- 4 pieces of flounder fillets
- 5 tablespoons vegetable oil /75ml

Instructions:

1) Place flounder fillets on a flat board, brush vegetable oil on the fillet using a cooking brush and then coat in bread crumbs.
2) Preheat the air fryer to 3900 F or 199°C .
3) Place the fillets in the double layer rack.
4) Cook for 15 minutes.
5) Serve and enjoy.

Nutrition information:

- Calories per serving: 277
- Carbs: 22.5g
- Protein: 26.9g
- Fat: 17.7g

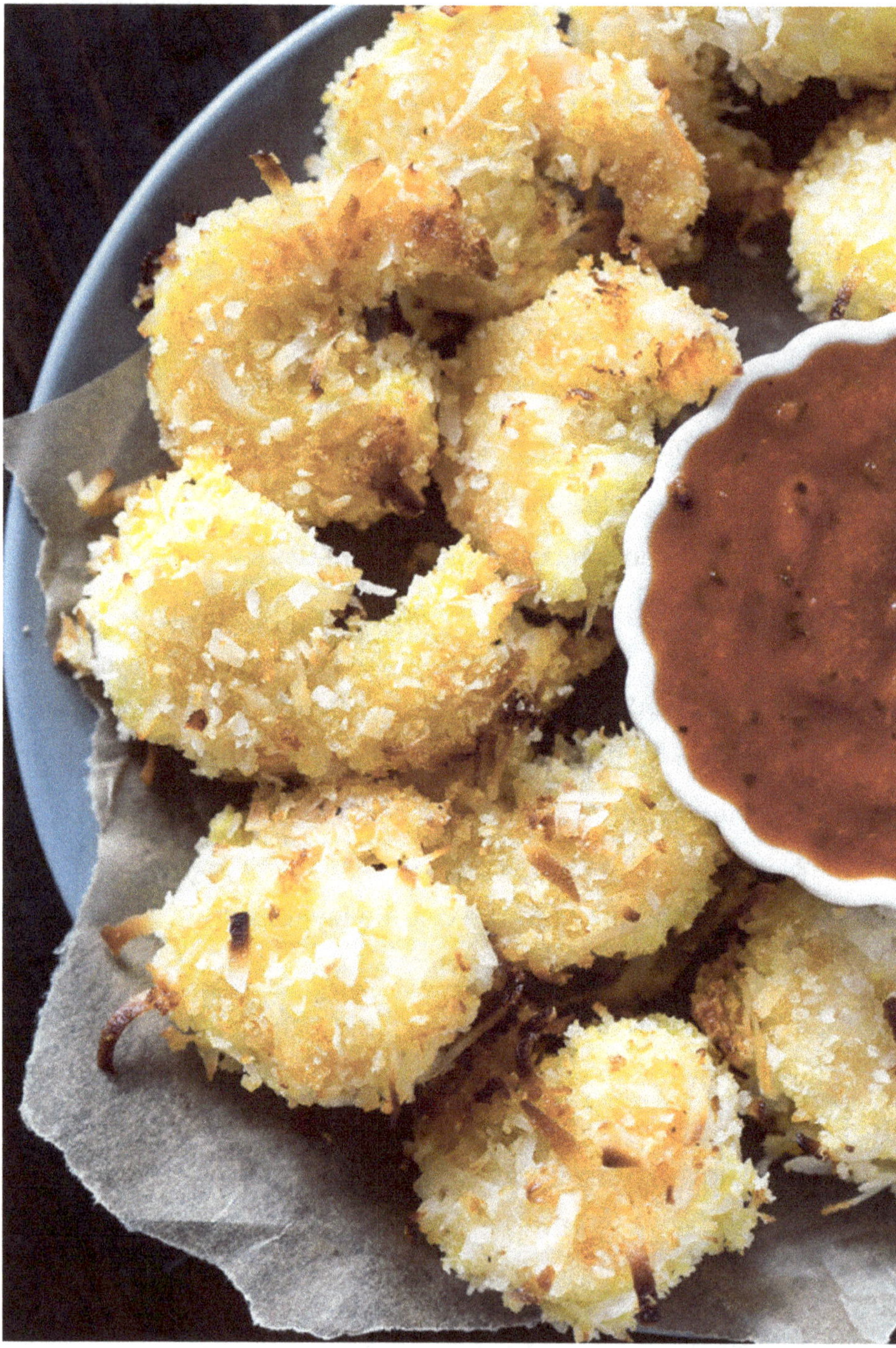

Crispy Coconut Covered Shrimps

Serves: 6

Cooking Time: 6 minutes

Ingredients:

- ½ cup almond flour /65g
- 1 cup dried coconut /130g
- 1 cup egg white
- 12 large shrimps, peeled and deveined
- 4 tablespoons butter /60g
- Salt and pepper to taste

Instructions:

1) Season the shrimps with salt and pepper to taste.
2) Place all ingredients in a very large Ziploc bag and shake well to combine.
3) Place the ingredients in an air fryer basket.
4) Cook for 6 minutes at 4000 F or 205°C .

Nutrition information:

- Calories per serving:272
- Carbohydrates:6.1g
- Protein: 15.3g
- Fat: 18.7g

Crispy Fish Fingers with Lemon-Garlic Herbs

Servings per Recipe: 1

Cooking Time: 10 minutes

Ingredients:

- ¼ teaspoon baking soda /1.25g
- ½ pound fish, cut into fingers /225g
- ½ teaspoon crushed black pepper /2.5g
- ½ teaspoon red chili flakes /2.5g
- ½ teaspoon salt /2.5g
- ½ teaspoon turmeric powder /2.5g
- 1 cup bread crumbs /130g
- 1 teaspoon ginger garlic paste /5g
- 2 eggs, beaten
- 2 tablespoons lemon juice /30ml
- 2 teaspoons cornflour /10g
- 2 teaspoons garlic powder /10g
- Oil for brushing

Instructions:

1) Preheat the air fryer to 3900 F or 199°C .
2) Season the fish fingers with salt, fresh lemon juice, turmeric powder, chili flakes, garlic powder, black

pepper, and garlic paste. Add the cornflour, eggs, and baking soda.

3) Heavily coat the seasoned fish in breadcrumbs and brush with olive oil.
4) Place on a double layer rack in the air fryer.
5) Cook for 10 minutes.

Nutrition information:

- Calories per serving: 773
- Carbs: 32.7g
- Protein: 64.9g
- Fat: 42.5g

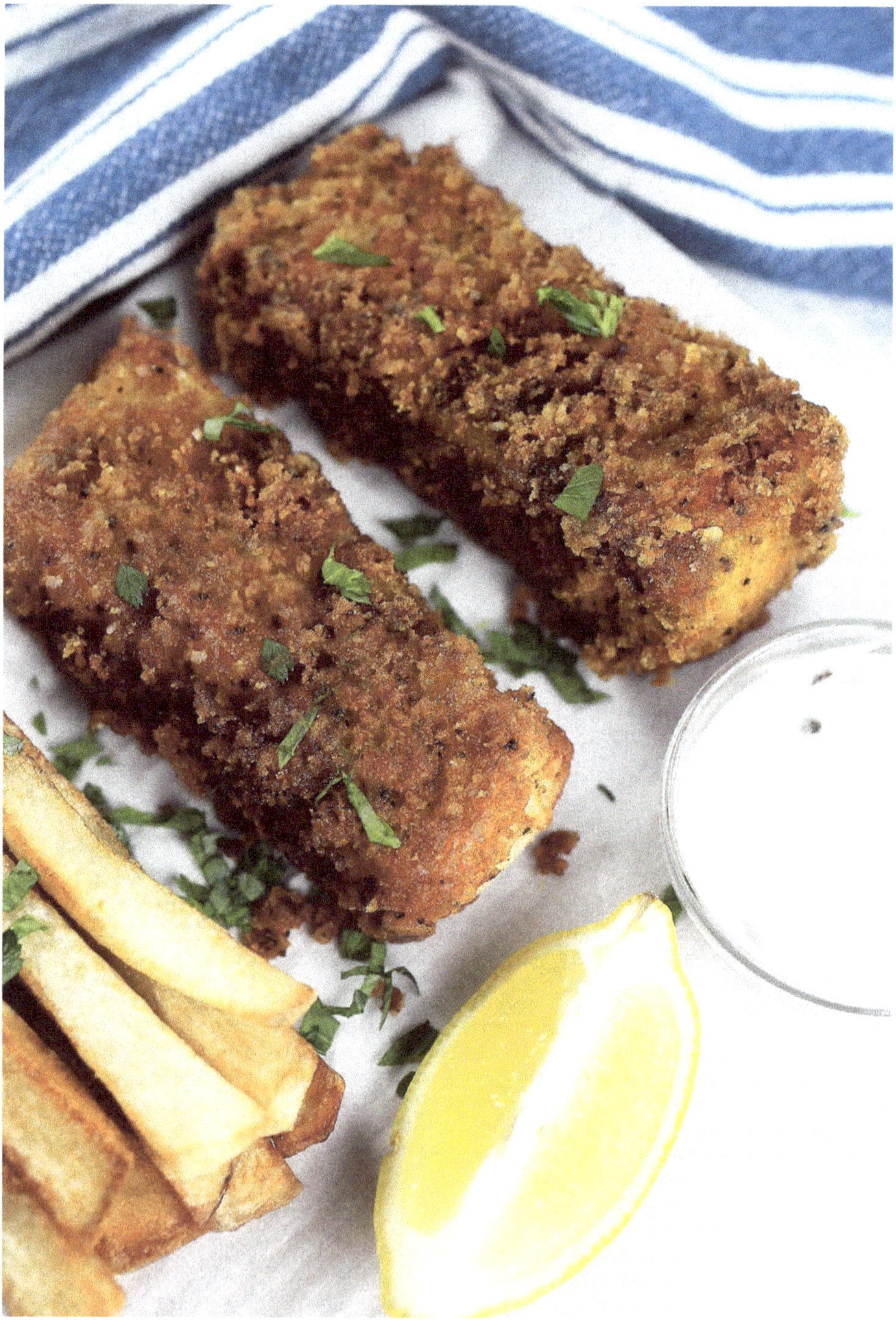

Crispy Fried Fish-Paprika Nuggets

Serves: 6

Cooking Time: 25 minutes

Ingredients:

- 1 ½ pounds fresh fish fillet, chopped finely/675g
- 1 cup almond flour /130g
- 1 tablespoon lemon juice /15ml
- 1 tablespoon olive oil /15ml
- 1 teaspoon chili powder /5g
- 1 teaspoon smoked paprika /5g
- 2 cloves of garlic, minced
- 2 eggs, beaten
- Salt and pepper to taste

Instructions:

1) Place all ingredients in a large bowl and mix well.
2) Use your hands to form small lumps. Place them in the fridge for two hours.
3) Preheat mid-air fryer for 5 minutes.
4) Carefully put the lumps in the air fryer basket.
5) Cook for 25 minutes at 3500 F or 177°C .

Nutrition information:

- Calories per serving: 359

- Carbohydrates: 21.7g
- Protein: 19.1g
- Fat: 21.7g

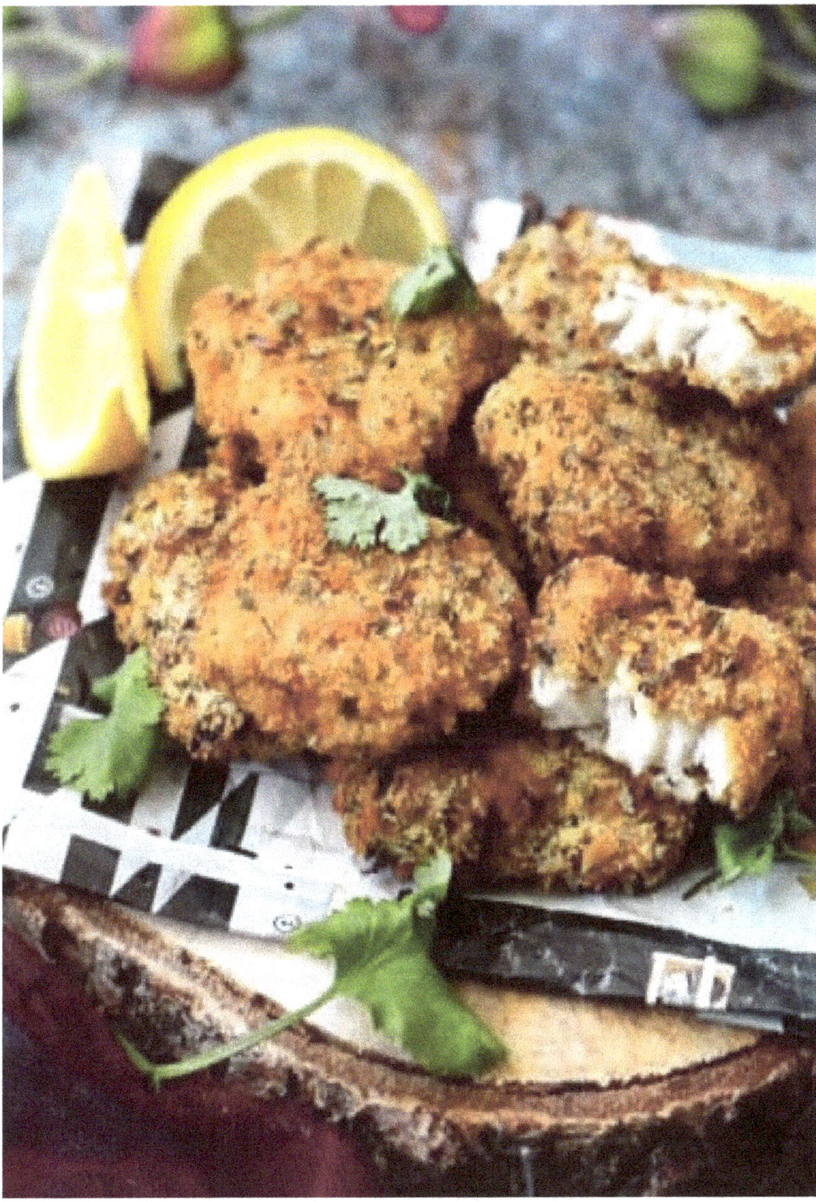

Crispy Lemon-Parsley Fish Cakes

Serves: 3

Cooking Time: 20 minutes

Ingredients:

- ½ cup dried coconut flakes /65g
- 1 cup almond flour /130g
- 1 cup cooked salmon, shredded /130g
- 1 tablespoon chopped parsley /15g
- 1 tablespoon freshly squeezed lemon juice /15ml
- 2 eggs, beaten
- 3 tablespoons coconut oil /45ml
- Salt and pepper to taste

Instructions:

1) Combine the salmon, almond flour, eggs, salt, pepper, fresh lemon juice and parsley in a large bowl. Form a thick dough.
2) Form small round balls with your hands and coat them in coconut flakes.
3) Brush the balls with coconut oil.
4) Preheat air fryer at 3250 F or 163°C .
5) Place the balls in a mid-air fryer basket and cook for 20 Minutes.

6) Shake the basket after 10 minutes of cooking.

Nutrition information:

- Calories per serving: 490
- Carbohydrates: 9.9g
- Protein: 35.5g
- Fat: 34.2g

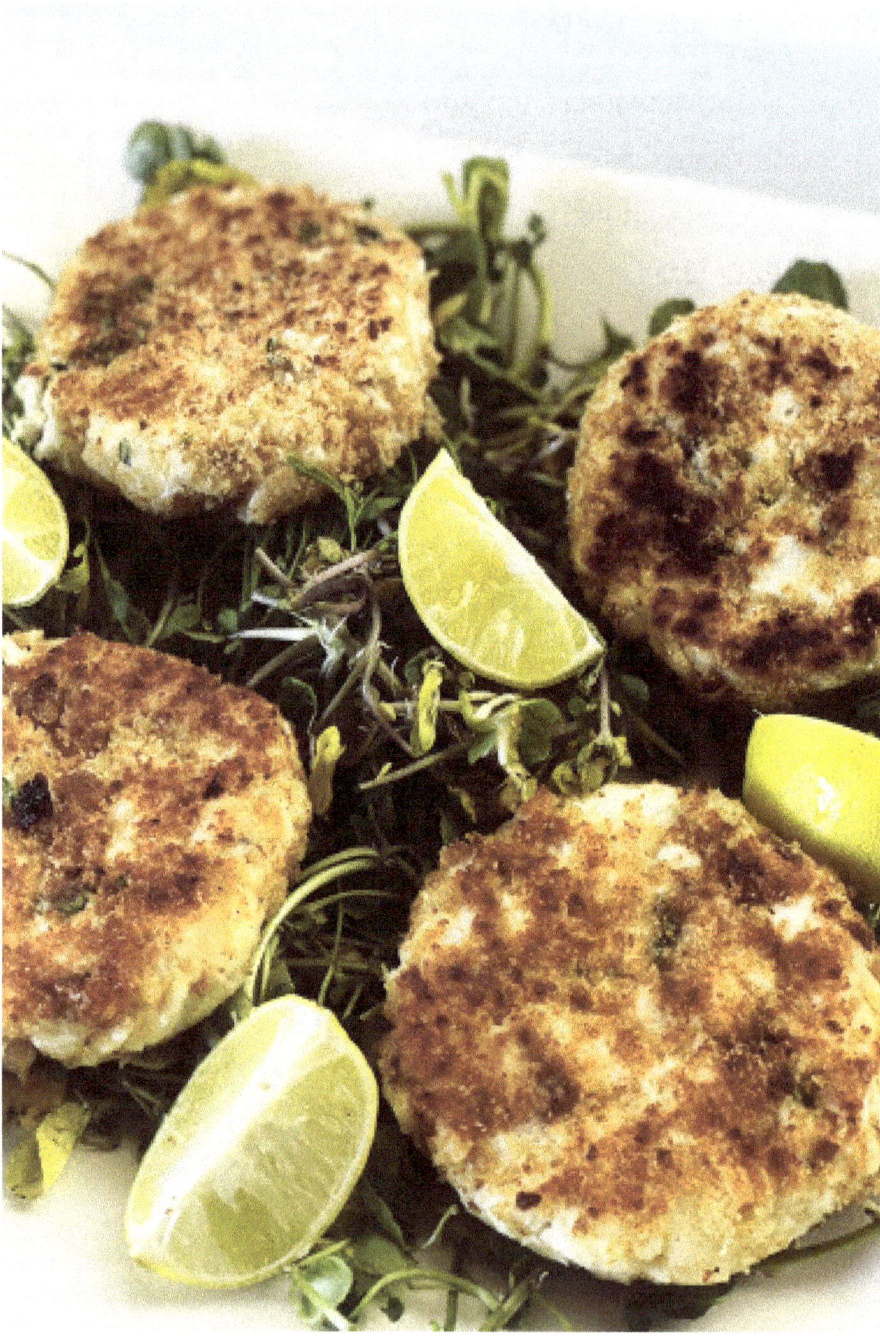

Crispy Shrimps the Cajun Way

Serves: 3

Cooking Time: 8 minutes

Ingredients:

- ¼ teaspoon red pepper cayenne /1.25g
- ¼ teaspoon smoked paprika /1.25g
- ½ pound tiger shrimps /2.5g
- ½ teaspoon old bay seasoning /2.5g
- 3 tablespoons olive oil /45ml
- A pinch of salt

Instructions:

1) Put on your air fryer and warm for 5 minutes.
2) Mix all ingredients in a bowl and then place the bowl in an air fryer.
3) Place the shrimps in a mid-air fryer basket and cook for 8 minutes at 3900 F or 199°C .

Nutrition information:

- Calories per serving: 213
- Carbohydrates: 0.3g
- Protein: 15.4g
- Fat: 16.7g

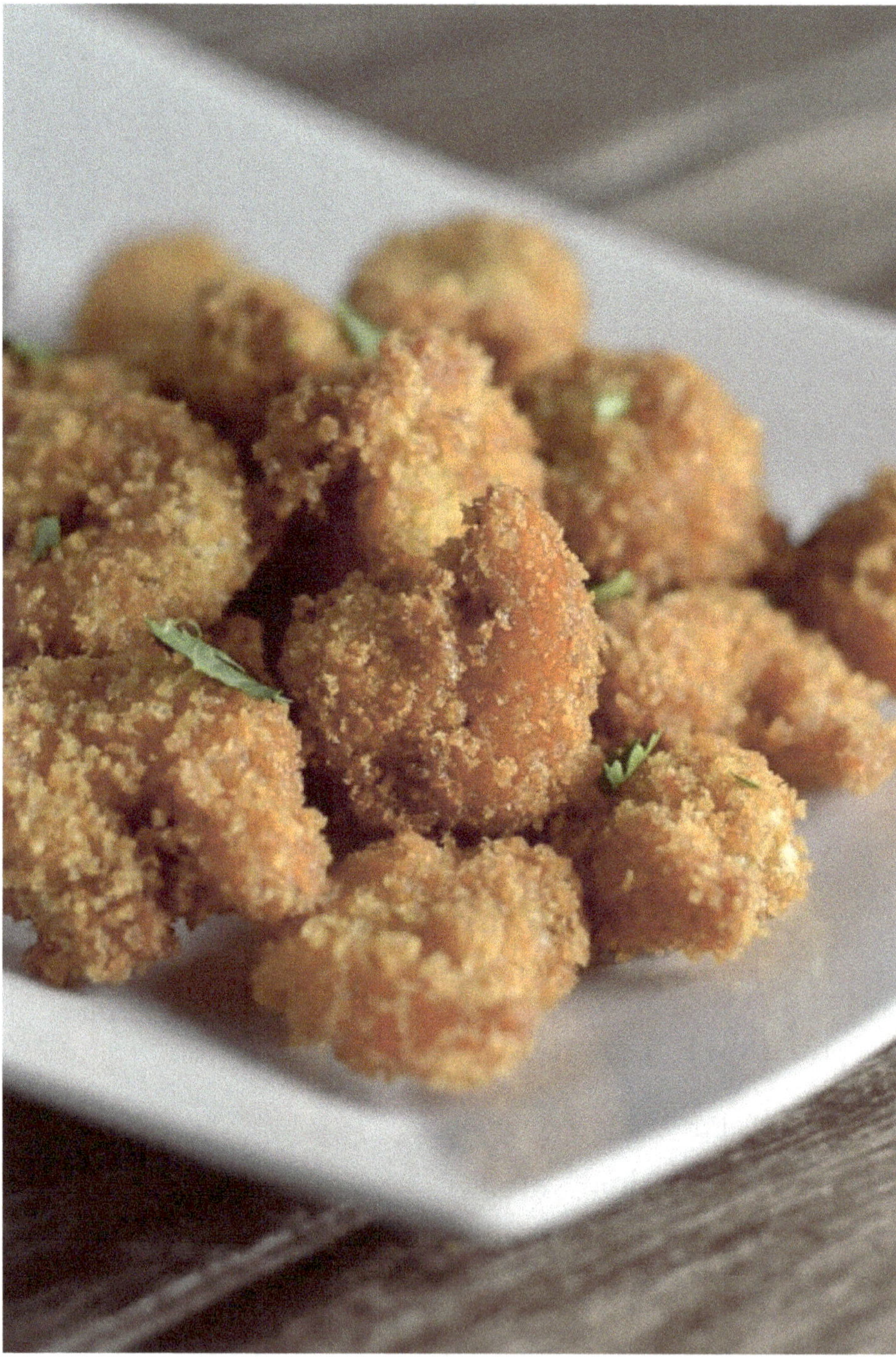

Crispy Spicy-Lime Fish Filet

Serves: 4

Cooking Time: 15

Ingredients:

- 1 egg white, beaten
- 1 tablespoon lime juice, freshly squeezed /15ml
- 1 teaspoon lime zest /5g
- 2 fish fillets, cut into pieces
- 2 tablespoons extra virgin olive oil /30ml
- 5 tablespoons almond flour /75g
- A dash of chili powder
- Salt and pepper to taste

Instructions:

1) Warm-up mid-air fryer for 5 minutes.
2) Place all ingredients in a Ziploc bag and shake until all ingredients are very well combined.
3) Place in the air fryer basket.
4) Cook for 15 minutes at 4000 F or 205°C .

Nutrition information:

- Calories per serving: 192
- Carbohydrates: 9.63g
- Protein: 8.14g

- Fat: 13.14g

Cumin, Thyme ‘n Oregano Herbed Shrimps

Servings per Recipe: 4

Cooking Time: 6 minutes

Ingredients:

- ¼ teaspoon red pepper cayenne /1.25g
- ¼ teaspoon red chili flakes /1.25g
- 1 teaspoon cumin /5g
- 1 teaspoon oregano /5g
- 1 teaspoon salt /5g
- 1 teaspoon thyme /5g
- 2 tablespoons coconut oil /30g
- 2 teaspoons cilantro /10g
- 2 teaspoons onion powder /10g
- 2 teaspoons smoked paprika /10g
- 20 jumbo shrimps, peeled and deveined

Instructions:

1) Preheat the air fryer to 3900 F or 199°C .
2) Season the shrimps with the Ingredients.
3) Place the seasoned shrimps within the double layer rack.
4) Cook for 6 minutes.

Nutrition information:

- Calories per serving: 220
- Carbs: 2.5g
- Protein: 34.2g
- Fat: 8.1g

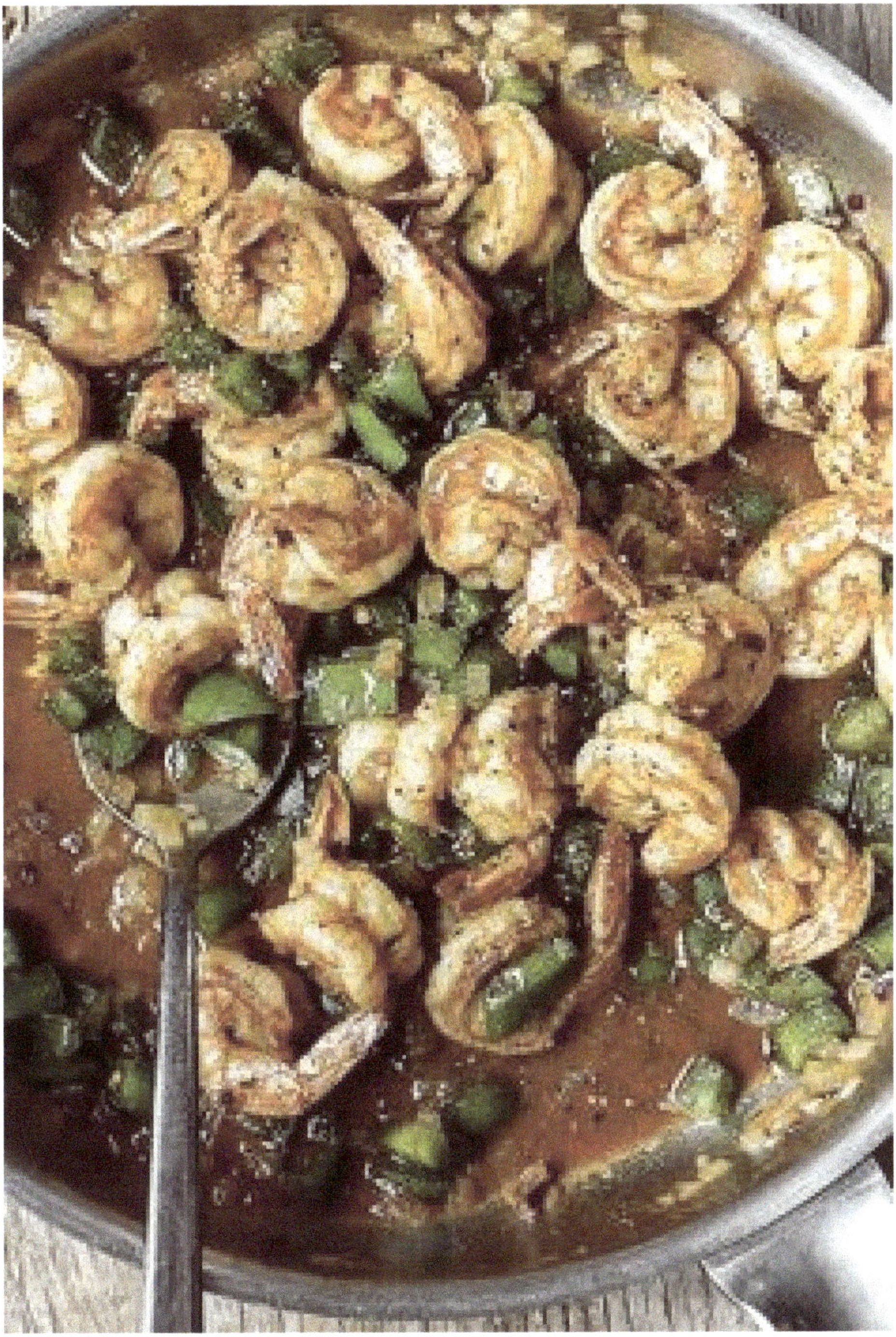

Crispy and Spicy Hot Shrimps

Serves: 6

Cooking Time: 5 minutes

Ingredients:

- ½ teaspoon ground black pepper /2.5g
- ½ teaspoon salt /2.5g
- 1 teaspoon chili flakes /5g
- 1 teaspoon chili powder /5g
- 12 fresh prawns, peeled and deveined
- 4 tablespoons essential olive oil /60ml

Instructions:

1) Warm up the air fryer for 5 minutes.
2) Find a bowl that can fit in your air fryer and mix all ingredients in it.
3) Place the shrimps in the air fryer basket and cook for 5 minutes at 4000 F or 205°C .

Nutrition information:

- Calories per serving: 156
- Carbohydrates: 0.8g
- Protein: 15.3g
- Fat: 10.2g

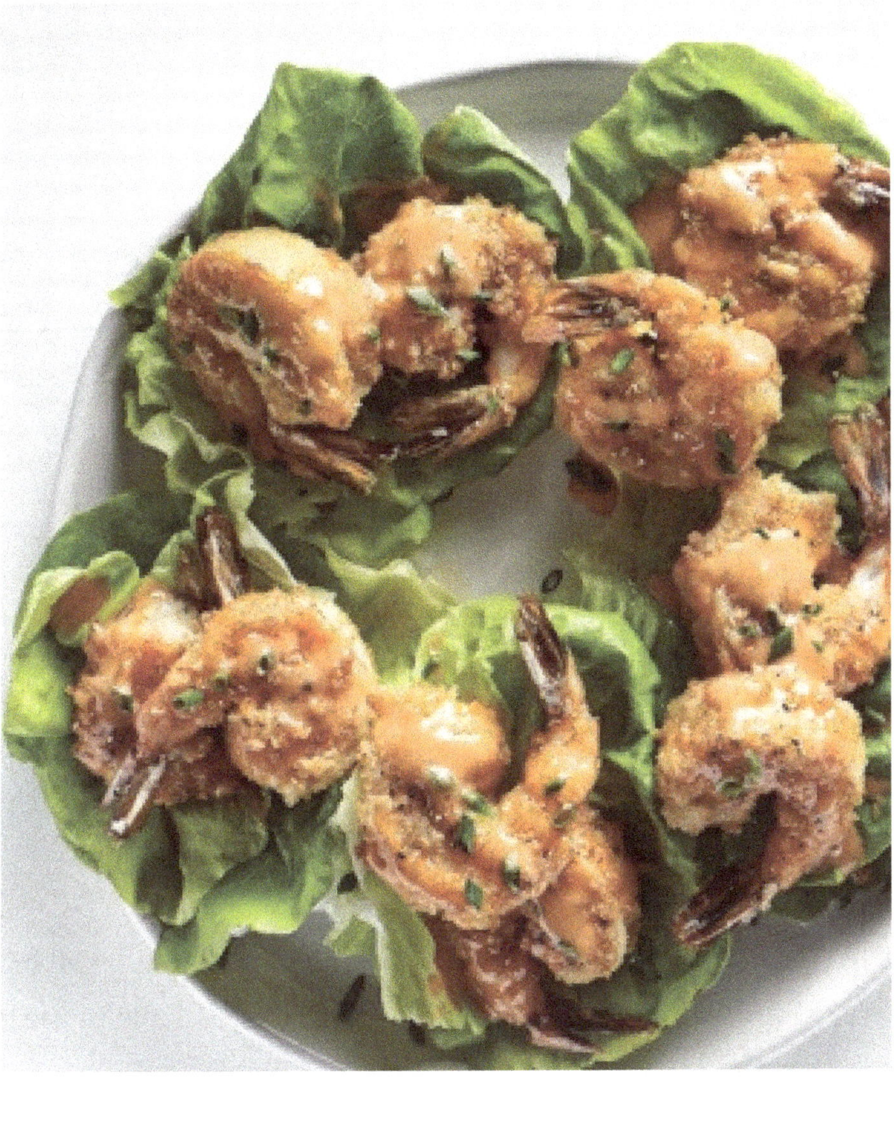

Dijon Mustard 'n Parmesan Crusted Tilapia

Servings per Recipe: 2

Cooking Time: 15

Ingredients:

1 tablespoon freshly squeezed lemon juice /15ml

1 teaspoon prepared horseradish /5g

1/4 cup dry bread crumbs /32.5g

2 tablespoons grated Parmesan cheese, divided /30g

2 teaspoons butter, melted /10ml

2 teaspoons Dijon mustard /10g

2 tilapia fillets (5 ounces each)

3 tablespoons reduced-fat mayonnaise /45ml

Instructions:

1) Sparingly grease baking pan of air fryer with any oil of your choice using a cooking spray. Place tilapia in the pan.
2) In a small bowl, whisk well mayo, fresh lemon juice, mustard, 1 tablespoon cheese and horseradish. Spread on the fish.

3) In another bowl, mix remaining cheese, melted butter, and bread crumbs. Sprinkle on the fish.
4) Cook for 15 minutes on 390 O F or 199°C .
5) Serve and enjoy.

Nutrition Information:

- Calories per Serving: 212
- Carbs: 7.0g
- Protein: 28.0g
- Fat: 8.0g

Drunken Skewered Shrimp, Tomatoes 'n Sausages

Servings per Recipe: 6

Cooking Time: 20 Minutes

Ingredients:

- 1/2 teaspoon dried crushed red pepper /2.5g
- 1/2 teaspoon freshly ground black pepper /2.5g
- 12 1-inch-long pieces andouille and another fully cooked smoked sausage
- 12 2-layer parts of red onion wedges
- 12 cherry tomatoes
- 12 uncooked extra-large shrimp (13 to 15 per pound), peeled, deveined
- 2 tablespoons chopped fresh thyme /30g
- 3/4 cup extra virgin olive oil /188ml
- 3/4 teaspoon salt /3.75g
- 4 large garlic cloves, pressed
- 4 teaspoons Sherry wine vinegar /20ml
- 5 teaspoons smoked paprika* /25g
- Nonstick vegetable oil spray

Instructions

1) Mix red pepper, black pepper, salt, wine vinegar, smoked paprika, thyme, garlic, and oil in a bowl. Transfer half into another bowl.
2) Fasten alternatively sausage and shrimp on steel skewers. Place skewers on the skewer rack in the air fryer and shower with all the paprika glaze. Cook in batches.
3) Allow cooking for 10 minutes at 3600 F or 183°C . After 5 minutes turn over skewers.
4) Serve with the dip kept aside.

Nutrition Information:

- Calories per Serving: 329
- Carbs: 9.8g
- Protein: 8.5g
- Fat: 28.4g

Easy 'n Crispy Cod Nuggets

Serves: 6

Cooking Time: 20 Minutes

Ingredients:

- ½ cup almond flour /65g
- 1 ½ pound cod fillet cut into big chunks /675g
- 1 egg, beaten
- 3 tablespoons olive oil /45ml
- Salt and pepper to taste

Instructions:

1) Warm up the air fryer for 5 minutes.
2) Season the cod fillets with salt and pepper to taste.
3) Add the eggs and stir to blend.
4) Coat the cod chunks in the almond flour and set them aside.
5) Brush the coated cod chunks with organic olive oil.
6) Place inside fryer basket and cook for 20 minutes at 3750 F or 191°C .

Nutrition information:

- Calories per serving: 170
- Carbohydrates: 0.9 g
- Protein: 18.2g

- Fat: 10.4g

Easy Battered Lemony Fillet

Serves: 4

Cooking Time: 15

Ingredients:

- ½ cup almond flour / 65g
- 1 egg, beaten
- 1 lemon
- 4 fish fillets
- 4 tablespoons vegetable oil /60ml
- Salt and pepper to taste

Instructions:

1) Spice the fish fillets with lemon, salt, and pepper to taste.
2) Dip the fish fillet in the beaten egg and then in almond flour, coat properly at all sides.
3) Place in mid-air fryer basket.
4) Cook for 15 minutes at 4000 F or 205°C .

Nutrition information:

- Calories per serving: 469
- Carbohydrates: 17.6g
- Protein: 15.8g
- Fat: 37.3g

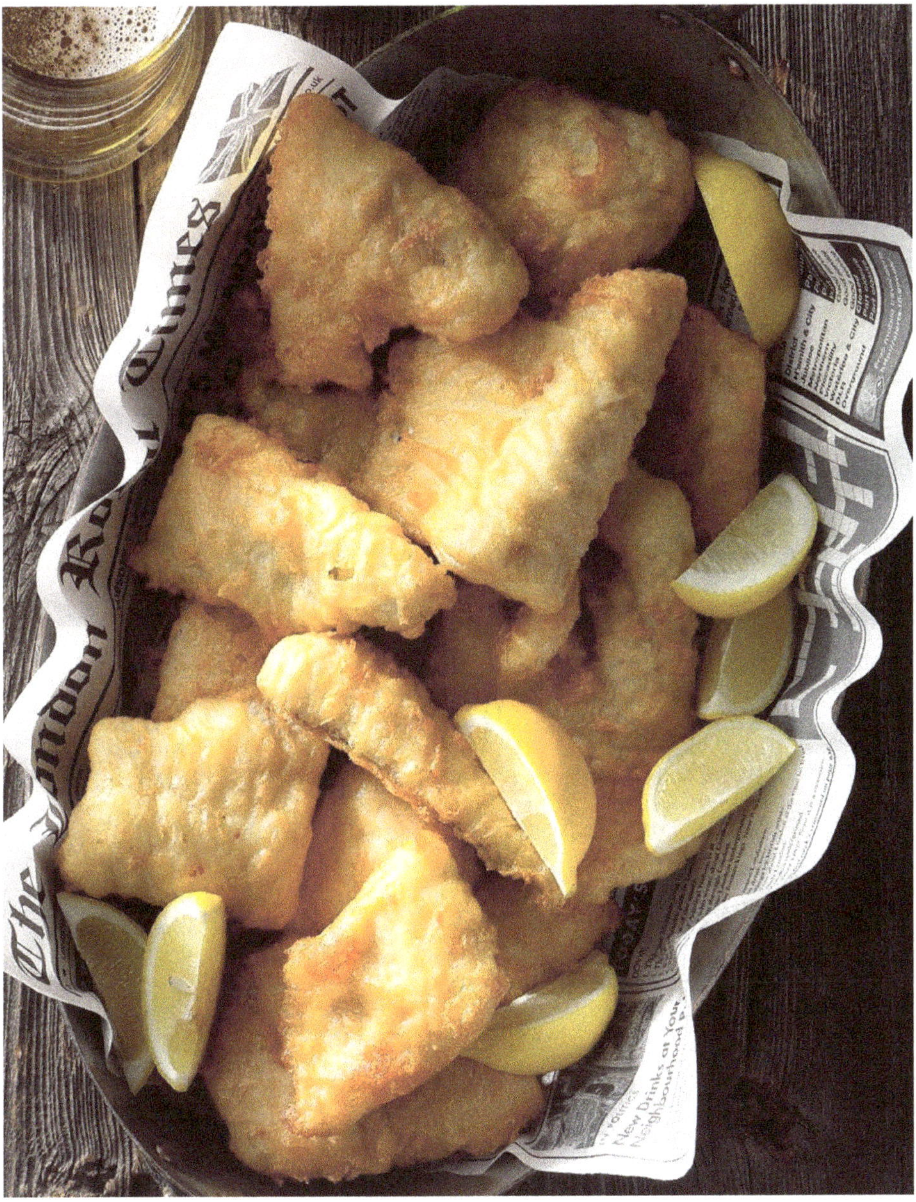

Easy Lobster Tail with Salted Butter

Servings per Recipe: 4

Cooking Time: 6 minutes

Ingredients:

- 2 tablespoons melted butter /30ml
- 4 lobster tails
- Salt and pepper to taste

Instructions:

1) Allow mid-air fryer to warm at 3900 F or 199°C .
2) Place the grill pan in the air fryer.
3) With scissors cut the lobster from the tail section.
4) Polish the lobster tails with melted butter and season with salt and pepper to taste.
5) Place in the grill pan and cook for 6 minutes.

Nutrition information:

- Calories per serving: 170
- Carbs: 1.1g
- Protein: 25.7g
- Fat: 6.9g

Easy Peasy Crispy Catfish Filet

Serves: 4

Cooking Time: 15

Ingredients:

- ¼ cup almond flour /32.5g
- 1 egg, beaten
- 4 catfish fillets
- 4 tablespoons organic olive oil /60ml
- Salt and pepper to taste

Instructions:

1) Warm up the air fryer for 5 minutes
2) Season the catfish fillets with salt and pepper to taste.
3) Dip in the beaten eggs and then coat in almond flour.
4) Polish the surface with olive oil
5) Place in the air fryer and cook for 15 minutes at 3500 F or 177°C .

Nutrition information:

- Calories per serving:308
- Carbohydrates: 1.3g
- Protein: 28.4g
- Fat: 20.6g

Egg Frittata with Smoked Trout

Serves: 6

Cooking Time: 15 minutes

Ingredients:

- 1 onion, chopped
- 2 fillets smoked trout, shredded
- 2 tablespoons coconut oil /60ml
- 2 tablespoons essential olive oil / 60ml
- 6 eggs, beaten
- ·Salt and pepper to taste

Instructions:

1) Allow the air fryer to preheat for 5 minutes.
2) Grab a mixing bowl, put all ingredients in it, and stir until well-combined.
3) Pour the above content into a baking pan.
4) Place in an air fryer and cook for 15 minutes at 4000 F or 205°C .

Nutrition information:

- Calories per serving: 254
- Carbohydrates: 3.4g
- Protein: 14.2g
- Fat:20.4g

Fennel Salad Topped with Roast Salmon

Servings per Recipe: 4

Cooking Time: 10 minutes

Ingredients:

- 1 clove of garlic, grated
- 1 teaspoon fresh thyme, chopped /5g
- 1 teaspoon salt /5g
- 2 tablespoons chopped dill /30g
- 2 tablespoons olive oil /30ml
- 2 tablespoons orange juice /30ml
- 2 teaspoons chopped parsley /30g
- 2/3 cup Greek yogurt /87g
- 4 pieces salmon fillets
- 4 cups sliced fennel /520ml

Instructions:

1) Preheat mid-air fryer to 3900 F or 199°C .
2) Season the salmon fillets with parsley, thyme, salt, and extra virgin olive oil.
3) Place the grill pan in the mid-air fryer.
4) Place the seasoned salmon fillet in the grill pan and cook for 10 minutes.
5) Turnover the fish halfway through cooking for even browning.

6) Mix the other ingredients in a bowl to make the salad.
7) Serve the fish with the salad.

Nutrition information:

- Calories per serving: 458
- Carbs: 9g
- Protein: 38g
- Fat: 30g

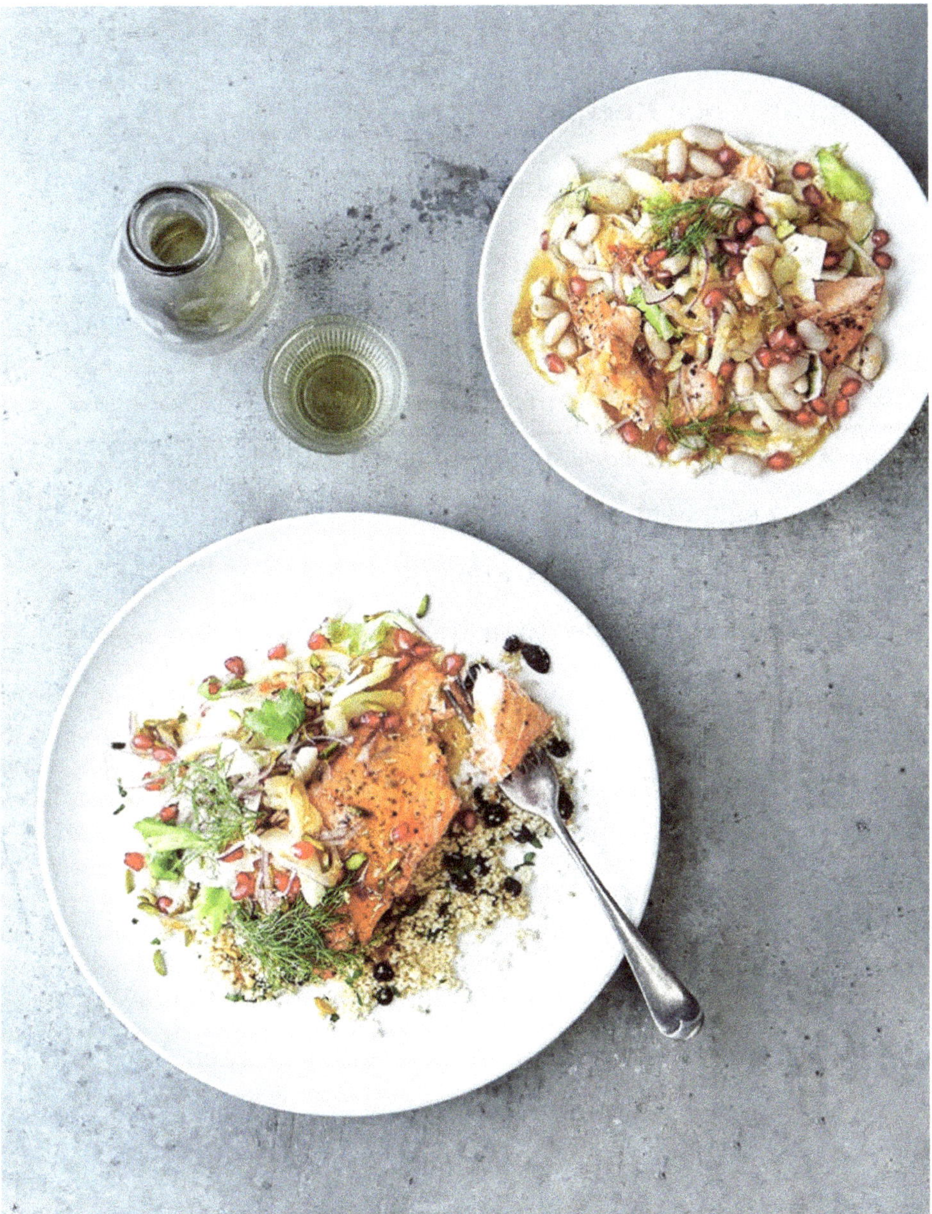

Fried Shrimps with Sweet Chili Sauce

Servings per Recipe: 1

Cooking Time: 6 minutes

Ingredients:

- ½ cup flour /65g
- ½ cup sweet chili sauce /125ml
- ½ pound raw shrimps, peeled and deveined /225g
- 1 egg, beaten
- 1 teaspoon chili powder /5g
- Salt and pepper to taste

Instructions:

1) Add shrimp and eggs to a large bowl, mix and season with salt and pepper to taste.
2) Mix chili powder and flour in another bowl.
3) Dip shrimps in flour mixture to coat.
4) Preheat mid-air fryer to 3300 F or 166°C .
5) Arrange shrimps on the double layer rack.
6) Cook for 6 minutes.
7) Serve with the schili sauce.

Nutrition information:

- Calories per serving: 719
- Carbs: 81.3g

- Protein: 66.4g
- Fat: 14.2g

Garlic-Cilantro Over Salmon Steak

Servings per Recipe: 2

Cooking Time: 15 minutes

Ingredients:

- ½ cup Greek yogurt /65g
- 1 cup cilantro leaves /130g
- 1 teaspoon honey /5g
- 2 cloves of garlic, minced
- 2 salmon steaks
- 2 tablespoons vegetable oil /30ml
- Salt and pepper to taste

Instructions:

1) Place the grill pan in the air fryer and preheat to 3900 F or 199°C .
2) Season the salmon steaks with salt and pepper and then brush with oil.
3) Grill for 15 minutes and flip over halfway through cooking.
4) In a blender, mix the garlic, cilantro leaves, yogurt and honey. Season with salt and pepper to taste. Pulse until smooth.
5) Serve the salmon steaks with all the cilantro sauce.

Nutrition information:

- Calories per serving: 485
- Carbs: 6.3g
- Protein: 47.6g
- Fat: 29.9g

Gingery Cod Filet Recipe from Hong Kong

Serves: 2

Cooking Time: 15

Ingredients:

- 2 cod fish fillets
- 250 mL water
- 3 tablespoons coconut aminos /45g
- 3 tablespoons coconut oil /45ml
- 5 slices of ginger
- A dash of sesame oil
- Green onions for garnish

Instructions:

1) Warm-up air fryer for 5 minutes.
2) Place all ingredients in a baking dish except the green onions.
3) Place in the air fryer and cook for 15 minutes at 4000 F or 205°C .
4) Dress with green onions.

Nutrition information:

- Calories per serving: 571
- Carbohydrates: 4.3g

- Protein: 22.3g
- Fat: 51.6g

Grilled Bacon 'n Scallops

Servings per Recipe: 2

Cooking Time: 12 minutes

Ingredients:

- 1 teaspoon smoked paprika /5g
- 6 bacon strips
- 6 large scallops

Instructions:

1) Wrap each bacon around a scallop and thread on a skewer.
2) Season with paprika.
3) Place on skewer rack in the air fryer.
4) Cook for 12 minutes at 3900 F or 199°C . Turnover skewers regularly while cooking.
5) Serve and enjoy.

Nutrition Information:

- Calories per Serving: 72
- Carbs: 2.4g
- Protein: 1.9g
- Fat: 6.0g

Grilled Scallops with Pesto

Servings per Recipe: 3

Cooking Time: 15

Ingredients:

- ½ cup prepared commercial pesto /45ml
- 12 large scallops, side muscles removed
- Salt and pepper to taste

Instructions:

1) Place all ingredients in a Ziploc bag. Place in a fridge to marinate for some hours.
2) Preheat air fryer to 3900 F or 199°C .
3) Place the grill pan in the air fryer.
4) Grill the scallops for 15 minutes.
5) Serve with pasta or bread (optional).

Nutrition information:

- Calories per serving: 137
- Carbs: 7.7g
- Protein:15.3 g
- Fat: 5g

Grilled Shrimp with Chipotle-Orange Seasoning

Servings per Recipe: 2

Cooking Time: 24 minutes

Ingredients:

- 3 tablespoons minced chipotles in adobo sauce/45ml
- salt
- ½-pound large shrimps /225g
- juice of 1/2 orange
- 1/4 cup barbecue sauce /62.5ml

Instructions

1) Mix all ingredients in a shallow bowl except the shrimp. Save one-quarter of the mixture for basting.
2) Add shrimp to a bowl and stir well to coat. Marinate for about 10 minutes.
3) Thread shrimps on skewers. Place on skewer rack in the air fryer.
4) Cook for 12 minutes at 3600 F or 183°C . Turnover skewers regularly while cooking. Also, saturate with sauce. If needed, cook in batches.
5) Serve and enjoy.

Nutrition Information:

- Calories per Serving: 179

- Carbs: 24.6g
- Protein: 16.6g
- Fat: 1.5g

Grilled Squid with Aromatic Sesame Oil

Servings per Recipe: 3

Cooking Time: 10 minutes

Ingredients:

- 1 ½ pounds squid, cleaned /675g
- 2 tablespoons toasted sesame oil /30ml
- Salt and pepper to taste

Instructions:

1) Preheat air fryer to 3900 F or 199°C .
2) Place the grill pan in the air fryer.
3) Season the squid with sesame oil, salt and pepper.
4) Grill the squid for 10 minutes.

Nutrition information:

- Calories per serving: 220
- Carbs: 0.9g
- Protein: 27g
- Fat: 12g

Healthy and Easy to Make Salmon

Servings per Recipe: 2

Cooking Time: 10

Ingredients:

- ½ of lemon
- 2 teaspoons avocado oil/10ml
- 2 teaspoons paprika/10ml
- 2 wild-caught salmon fillets
- Salt and pepper to taste

Instructions:

1) Preheat air fryer to 3900 F or 199°C .
2) Season the salmon fillets with avocado oil, paprika, salt, and pepper, then sprinkle with lemon juice on both sides.
3) Place the grill pan in a mid-air fryer.
4) Place the salmon fillets in the grill pan and cook for 10 Minutes.
5) Turn over the fillets to the other side halfway through the cooking time.

Nutrition information:

- Calories per serving: 382
- Carbs: 2.2g
- Protein: 66.1g

- Fat: 12g

Honey-Ginger Soy Sauce Over Grilled Tuna

Servings per Recipe: 3

Cooking Time: 20 Minutes

Ingredients:

- 1 ½ pounds tuna, thick slices /675g
- 1 serrano chili, seeded and minced
- 2 tablespoons grated fresh ginger /30g
- 2 tablespoons honey /30g
- 2 tablespoons peanut oil /30ml
- 2 tablespoons rice vinegar /30ml
- 2 tablespoons soy sauce /30ml

Instructions:

1) Place all ingredients in a Ziploc bag.
2) Allow to marinate inside the fridge for some hours.
3) Preheat the air fryer to 3900 F or 199°C .
4) Place the grill pan in the air fryer.
5) Grill the fish for 15 to 20 Minutes.
6) Turnover the fish halfway through the cooking time to achieve uniform browning.
7) Meanwhile, place the marinade in a saucepan and allow to boil gently for 10 minutes before it thickens.

8) Brush the sides of the tuna with all the sauce before serving.

Nutrition information:

- Calories per serving: 357
- Carbs:14.8 g;
- Protein: 44.9g
- Fat: 13.1g

Jamaican-Jerk Seasoned Salmon

Servings per Recipe: 2

Cooking Time: 12 minutes

Ingredients:

- 1 ½ tablespoons mayonnaise /22.5ml
- 1 teaspoon grated lime zest /5g
- 1/4 cup sour cream /62.5ml
- 1/4 cup sweetened shredded coconut, toasted /32.5g
- 2 salmon fillets (6 ounces or 180geach)
- 2 teaspoons Caribbean jerk seasoning /10g
- 4 tbsp cream of coconut /60ml
- 4 tbsp cup lime juice /60ml

Instructions:

1) Lightly spray the baking pan with oil. Place the salmon in the baking pan.
2) Cook for 12 minutes at 3300 F or 166°C .
3) Place pan over medium heat. Add lime juice, lime zest, cream of coconut, and sour cream and allow to simmer. Stir continuously. Allow to cool and pour the content in a bowl for dipping.
4) Serve and enjoy.

Nutrition Information:

- Calories per Serving: 490
- Carbs: 16.0g
- Protein: 30.0g
- Fat: 34.0g

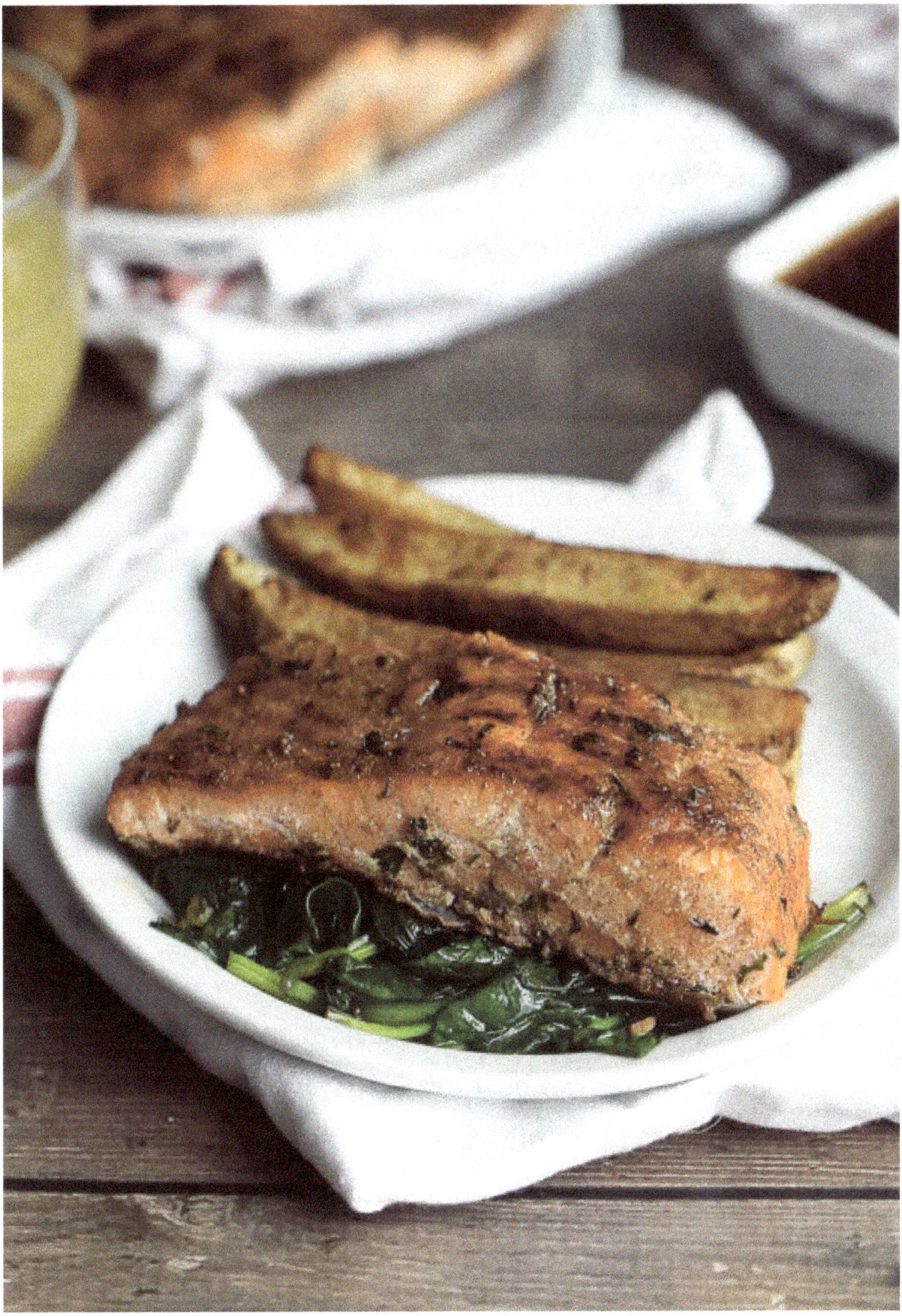

Lemon Tuna 'n Buttered Rice Puff

Servings per Recipe: 6

Cooking Time: 60 Minutes

Ingredients:

- 1 teaspoon salt /5g
- 2 egg yolks1 (12 ounces or /360g) can tuna, undrained
- 2 tablespoons grated onion /30g
- 1 tablespoon fresh lemon juice /15ml
- 2 egg whites
- 1 1/2 cups milk /375ml
- 1 1/3 cups water /333ml
- 1/3 cup butter /30ml
- 1/4 cup all-purpose flour /43g
- 1/4 teaspoon ground black pepper /1.25
- 2/3 cup uncooked white rice /87g

Instructions:

1) Bring water to boil in a saucepan and add in the rice. Cook under low heat until rice is cooked. This usually takes about 20 minutes.
2) Melt butter in another saucepan over medium heat. Add in pepper, salt, and flour. Stir until completely combined. Cook for two minutes. Slowly add milk while stirring continuously. Keep at it until thickened.

3) Whisk egg yolks in a medium-sized bowl. While whisking slowly pour this mixture in the thickened milk mixture and continue cooking and stirring for 2 more minutes while you add lemon juice, onion, tuna, and rice.
4) Sparingly grease the baking pan with cooking spray. And pour in the rice mixture.
5) Whisk egg whites well and slowly add to the rice mixture.
6) Cover the pan with a foil.
7) Cook for 20 minutes at 3600 F or 183°C until the top is lightly brown and the middle is done.
8) Serve and enjoy.

Nutrition Information:

- Calories per Serving: 302
- Carbs: 24.1g
- Protein: 20.6g
- Fat: 13.6g

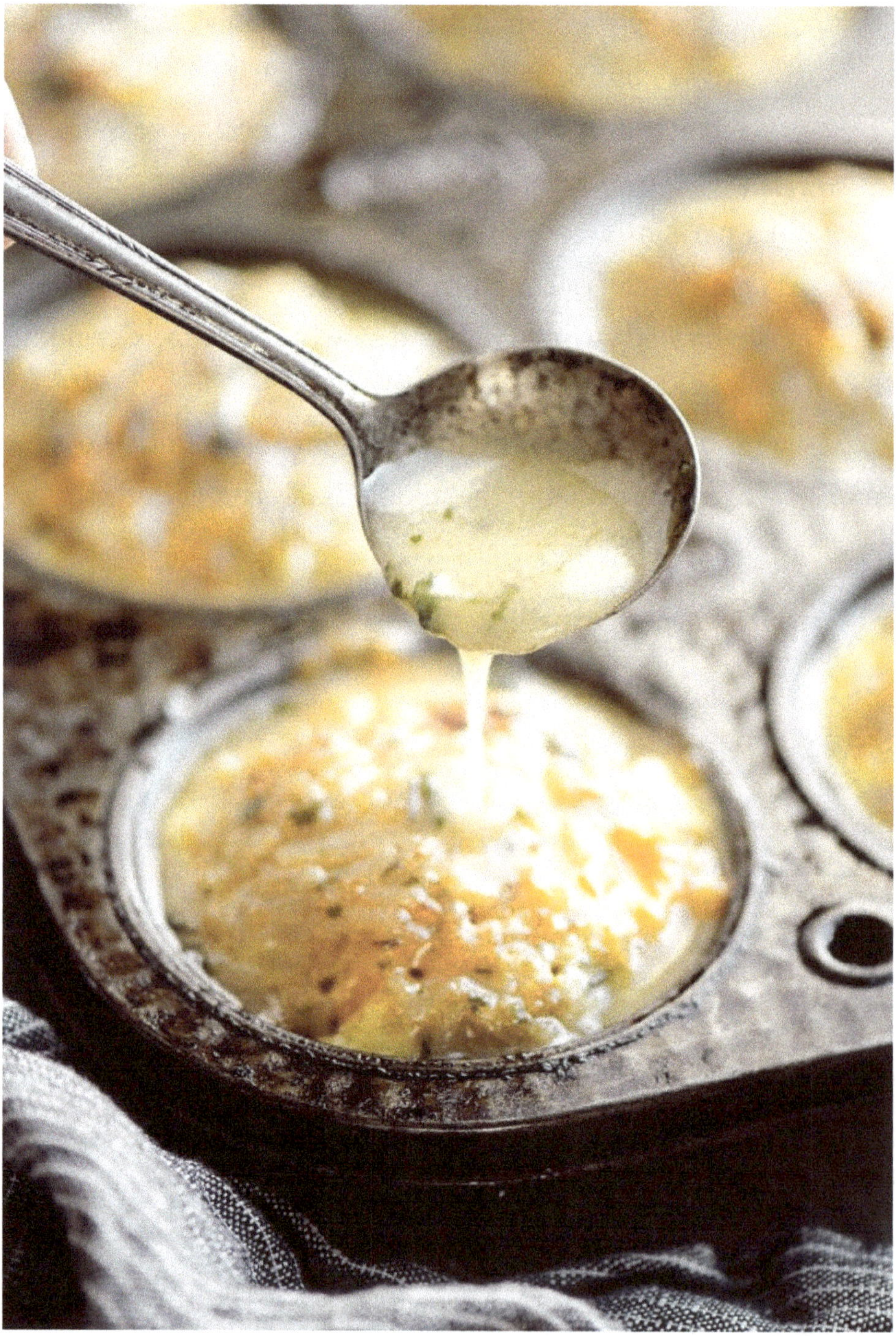

CPSIA information can be obtained
at www.ICGtesting.com
Printed in the USA
BVHW061942150621
609630BV00003B/306

9 781803 172361